PICASSO'S
WOMAN

PICASSO'S WOMAN

A Breast Cancer Story

Rosalind MacPhee

Douglas & McIntyre
Vancouver/Toronto

For Peter, Katherine and Jenny,
who put so much loving energy behind me,
and did so much more

94 95 96 97 98 5 4 3 2 1

Douglas & McIntyre
1615 Venables Street
Vancouver, British Columbia   V5L 2H1

Canadian Cataloguing in Publication Data

MacPhee, Rosalind, 1946-
  Picasso's woman

  ISBN 1-55054-158-7

  1. MacPhee, Rosalind, 1946-   2. Breast—Cancer—Patients—
Biography.   I. Title.
RC280.B8M32 1994   362.1'9699449'0092   C94-910606-2

Editing by Barbara Pulling
Cover design by Tania Craan
Cover illustration by Barbara Klunder
Typeset by Brenda and Neil West, Typographics West
Printed and bound in Canada by D. W. Friesen & Sons Ltd.
Printed on acid-free paper ∞

The publisher gratefully acknowledges the assistance of the Canada Council and the British Columbia Ministry of Tourism, Small Business, and Culture for its publishing programs.

Some of the proceeds from the sales of this book will be donated to the Canadian Breast Cancer Foundation.

"The world breaks every one and afterward
many are strong at the broken places."

ERNEST HEMINGWAY

A Farewell to Arms

Acknowledgements

I have never before written anything as personal as *Picasso's Woman*. Although I have made every effort to be true to the experience, I know that each person in this book could tell his or her own version of the story. For narrative purposes, I have done some telescoping of time and focussed on events that best serve the spirit of the book. Names have been changed in several instances.

My breast cancer was diagnosed early in 1991. Without the loving support of many people, this account of what can happen to even a determinedly optimistic person could never have been written. Special thanks to my friend Deirdre, who gave much of herself by allowing me to write about a time that was difficult for us both. Thanks also to my remarkable friend Pat for standing on chairs and cheering my every effort. I am indebted to the following people, who not only believed in the importance of this work but loaned me secluded places in which to write: Jocelyn and Ken Steuart, Jacki and Sandy Jamieson, Goldie and Paul Charles, Joan and Rob Lemmers, the Whitelaw and Fedoruk families, Elaine Stevens, Marilyn and Stewart Blusson, Sally and Doug Pollock, Annie Arstall and Wayne Smith. I'd also like to give my thanks to Joanna Anthony, Diane Bergeron, Sue Cameron, Des Loan, Gillian and Douglas Miller, Dr. Ivo Olivotto, Cheryl Smith, Mike Yates, the Charles and Kincade families, and my co-workers with the ambulance service. To all my friends, a heartfelt thank you.

I am grateful to Douglas & McIntyre for approaching me to write this book and for their continued interest and enthusiasm. For her gently questioning, insightful and supportive readings of my manuscript, I am indebted to my gifted editor, Barbara Pulling. I thank my agent, Denise Bukowski, for recognizing the need for such a work. Keith Maillard was responsible for prodding me to write the original essay.

The women at the Canadian Breast Cancer Foundation have been a real source of inspiration. I am grateful to Judy Caldwell for writing the all-important Afterword. The countless cancer patients I have known in recent years have instilled in me an unwavering sense of purpose. I wish in particular to remember Ellen Pareis, Shannon Tayata, Virginia Whitelaw and Allana Wight.

1

I'VE ALWAYS LIKED ADVENTURES. Adventures are about being brave, fighting back, and keeping your wits about you. Adventures are about taking control. Survival. I believe that, in any adventure, who people are can be determined not by what happens to them but by how they deal with it.

The small village where I live, a forty-five-minute drive from downtown Vancouver, provides a natural setting for adventure. My husband, Peter, and I drove the famously dangerous Sea to Sky Highway over Bailey bridges and washed-out creeks more than twenty years ago to buy a piece of wilderness on a forty-degree slope, and that says something about us both, I suppose. The community of Lions Bay had a long history of landslides at the time; the mountainside around it periodically let go its terrible tonnage, taking out everything in its path all the way down to the ocean.

The local place names reveal much about what Lions Bay is like today: Unnecessary Mountain, Lone Tree Creek, Yahoo Tunnel, Daybreak Point, Whale Rock, Lookout Point. So do the names of the streets: Oceanview, Isleview, Mountainview, Sunset, Crosscreek, Tidewater, Timbertop. Not so long ago, two nearby mountains were christened Thomas and David in memory of two local youths who were buried under one of the massive slides.

The house my husband and I built, where we now live with our two teen-aged daughters, is a hidden, secret place. Set deep in West Coast rain forest, it is approached by a long driveway that stops at the bottom of a series of flights of steps. We believed, naively perhaps, that the daily hike up stairs through forest to our front entrance would keep us young—in fact, my husband once calculated that I climb Mount Everest twice a year just to bring in the groceries and walk the dog. We retained the surrounding forest not only because we love trees but also for reasons of privacy; our neighbours' houses—a hundred feet to the north and to the south—are scarcely visible.

As newlyweds, Peter and I weren't sure what to do with our half-acre of steep slope, so we hired an architect who had been influenced by indigenous wood structures such as barns, mineshafts, canneries and the cedar dwellings of the Haida. Our home has elements of all these structures: it's a do-it-yourself, board-by-board project that started off as a five-year plan and still has not been completed.

We have always thought of our unfinished piece of heaven on earth as a project in treehouse living. The tall, weathered house appears to rise organically from the land. The rear is set into a fern-covered slope; the front offers a through-the-trees view of distant islands and ocean. There is a beauty that needs to be understood in mathematical terms of volumes, angles and planes—in design, the house is a cube cut off at a forty-five-degree angle, providing a southwest exposure for almost all the windows. The interior has four open split-level floors above a basement. The master bedroom level, at the top, overlooks the study, dining room and kitchen. The kitchen level overlooks the living room, which in turn overlooks our daughters' bedrooms. A central open staircase serves as the means of flow from one level to the next. Cathedral-like, the exposed cedar ceiling of skylights and rafters is angled towards the sky. When light streams through the high vertical windows, it's a spiritual happening.

Adventure is something I've gone to great lengths to bring into my daily life. Under the pretence of doing research for a book of poetry, I hiked the Chilkoot Pass from Alaska to British Columbia and paddled a canoe down six hundred miles of wilderness to Dawson City in the Yukon. The truth is, I wrote the book so that I'd have an excuse to be off on my own in the North. I helped set up a search and rescue team in Lions Bay—if nothing else was going on, there was always the possibility of searching the local mountains for some lost soul. I got high on the metaphysics of writing, climbed narrow mountain trails to photograph hanging lakes and alpine meadows, fished from my kayak. My profession as a paramedic offered me an ever-changing world; it was a job that often instructed me to abandon any illusion of control over my fate. Attending university as a part-time student gave me the opportunity to investigate a variety of fields. At a time when I was preoccupied with little more than studying the history of art, I became involved in an unexpected turn of events.

This particular adventure started on an ice-cold, rainy January day with high winds. Nothing to bring down trees, but enough to lure me to the ocean with its impossible swells. Breakers thundered onto my kayak, the horizon rising and dipping as I paddled madly between waves high enough to block my view of the mountains. I arrived home exhilarated but, like the Anglo-Saxon seafarer, cold wrapped and bound in frost.

In the shower I thought, What's this? At first I didn't pay much attention to what felt like a lump in one of my breasts. I'd never been overly concerned with my physical appearance, and I was terribly offhand about anything that happened within my body. I assumed that if I ignored whatever seemed to be wrong the problem would disappear as mysteriously as it had appeared.

But with the warm water pouring over me, I gave some thought to the sharp little pains in my right breast that I'd more or less ignored for about a month. On the occasions when I'd ignored these pains *less*, my mind had entertained the possibilities. I had read an article about breast cancer that said a malignant lump is normally asymptomatic: if it hurts, it's probably not cancer. The abnormality I'd just found felt hard. And it hurt. Now I admitted to myself, reluctantly, that it had been hurting with increasing intensity for some time.

My fingers returned obsessively to my breast, hoping that the lump would somehow be gone. But each time, I was startled by how enormous it felt. How could I possibly have missed it before this? I assured myself that it must be the fibrocystic change that some women get just before their periods. I thought back to conversations with friends who had been troubled by painful, lumpy breasts. I wished I had paid more attention. Something about too much coffee. Something about Vitamin E.

After I had dried off, I stood naked before a mirror. Amazingly, the lump was not visible. I stared at the rest of my body, looking for signs of malignancy everywhere. Although nothing was noticeably different, I was overwhelmed by the feeling that something was wrong. I went to the kitchen and poured myself some coffee, noticing that my mug was half empty before I even sat down.

The lump had turned up during a period of my life when I felt a kinship with Superwoman—I seemed to have the uncanny ability to stretch time. I successfully juggled my roles as wife and mother, paramedic and station chief, poet and student about to complete my Fine Arts degree. Somehow, I still managed to make time for the pleasures of kayaking, hiking and socializing with friends. But no matter how hard I tried to push my fears to the back of my mind, my job as a paramedic had taught me that lightning likes to strike something. A week after discovering the lump, I talked myself into having it checked by a doctor.

January was warming slightly, but the rain had gathered into a steady downpour the day I went to see Duncan, our family doctor. The nurse and I exchanged small talk about the latest deluge. Then she handed me a gown and left, saying cheerily, "Everything off, dear."

Duncan greeted me warmly, pointing out that it was almost three years since I'd had a physical.

"Ah, yes, but here I am," I replied, saying nothing about the lump.

He was casual but methodical in his examination. When he checked my breasts, I began to perspire. He was very thorough, checking first the left breast, then the right. He finished the exam, then turned to pick up my file. "Okay," he said. "Everything looks good."

My first inclination was to flee. A reprieve, I thought. But something held me back.

I was amazed at how casual my voice sounded. "Could you check the right breast again? I think there's a lump of some sort there."

He palpated the upper part of my breast again, firmly but gently. "Where exactly have you felt it?"

I stared at the wall, focussing on a photograph of a church with a lopsided bell-tower. "At about five o'clock," I told him.

His experienced fingers moved around my breast, and then his hand stopped. "Here?"

"Yes."

I looked at his eyes, trying to gauge his response, but he remained professionally cool. "There's certainly something here, isn't there?"

"What do you think it is?"

"I don't know ... probably a cyst."

He washed his hands in a small sink and continued talking. "There are two approaches we can take—you can come back in a couple of weeks so we can catch it in a different phase of your menstrual cycle, or you can be referred to a specialist right away."

He drew a picture of my breast in my file, dividing the diagram into four quadrants. He added a crude circle for the lump and wrote down approximate dimensions. Without stopping the motion of his pen, he asked, "Do you have any feelings about what you'd like to do?"

"Get rid of it?" I smiled, uncertainly.

"I can understand that ... but remember that 80 per cent of the time, these masses don't amount to anything."

"Well, I've already been coexisting with this *thing* for a while. I'd like to know what it is."

"Fair enough. Do you have anyone you'd like to be referred to?"

"No. Who's the best?"

"Dr. Harris. He's an excellent surgeon."

I tried not to zero in on the word "surgeon." "He's good with his hands?"

"Yes, but as I said, you probably have a cyst. Dr. Harris will draw the fluid off through a needle and bingo—your lump will be gone."

I folded the referral slip into my pocket. I heard him say, "I'd also like you to have another mammogram."

"Actually, I've never had one."

"Never?"

I shook my head slowly.

He looked worried. "Haven't I asked you?"

"Well, yes, you have. I've taken the slips home, but I've never gotten around to making the appointments."

"Why?"

"Probably because I've always felt I'd die from falling off a mountain or rolling my kayak one time too many, long before any disease would ever get me."

"Well, this is one mammogram I want you to have," he said. "And I'd like to see you again about a week after you see the surgeon."

I dressed and walked out into a day that remained cheerless and rainy. From a telephone booth, I dialled the specialist's number and explained my referral to his nurse. Today was Wednesday. While she left me on hold, I wondered how many months it would be before I was able to see the doctor.

"Ms MacPhee?" her voice sang pleasantly. "Dr. Harris can see you at two o'clock on Tuesday afternoon." I was surprised and disconcerted.

It wasn't so easy to book an appointment for a mammogram; the first available time was two weeks away. I fought off the thought that I had let myself down. What if the mammogram showed a mass that could have been detected a long time ago? Like everyone, I'd heard the slogan: "Find it early—cancer can be beaten."

The rain had eased off to a drizzle, and I decided to go for a walk along the ocean. I worked hard at convincing myself that the lump was nothing, fighting off a feeling in my body that something was very wrong. I was overreacting, I told myself. Nothing had been diagnosed. Fibrocystic lumps come and go.

Cancer was someone else's problem. I was much too healthy to have it.

I did know from my work as a paramedic that breast cancer was a disease on the rise, and one that struck many thousands of women. I knew that in North America one woman in nine could expect to be diagnosed with the disease. I'd even read some reports saying one woman in eight. Although I had heard of wonderful new discoveries and treatments, I also knew that the diagnosis meant imminent death to a great number of people. Many of the patients I saw were in very advanced stages of breast cancer. To them, I must have seemed like the indestructible woman. At that moment, as I walked along the edge of the water, I didn't feel very indestructible. I felt cold and alone. And frightened.

When I opened the front door, I was greeted enthusiastically by our dog, Freyja. Freyja is a harlequin Great Dane—harlequin describes not only her patches of black and white but also her clownish nature. She is such a focus for our family that we sometimes call ourselves "Freyja's people." Today, as any other day, Freyja had no time for my preoccupations. She demanded attention, and lots of it.

I fixed her dinner, then scanned the shelves of books that lined the living room walls. I was looking for the medical reference work my family had always jokingly called the *Cancer Book*. A few nosebleeds? Probably cancer. Dizzy spells at the height of summer? Cancer. Headaches? Probably only a few days left to live.

Cancer, the book informed me, is "the unregulated, disorganized proliferation of cell growth capable of killing the host by the spread of cells from the site of origin to distant sites, or by local spread." It went on to explain that the word meant anything bad or harmful that spreads and destroys. Then I saw the line I dreaded: "Cancer leads through definite stages to death."

Suddenly feeling weak, I lay down. A small fire was still burning in the cast iron woodstove at the head of the sofa. At the other end of the long cedar room was a grand piano with a gleaming trumpet lying on top. The firelight flickered on everything in between: Inuit prints, books, snowshoes, kayak paddles, fishing rods, climbing gear, cameras and pottery, along with a variety of boots and jackets by the door.

I stared at the books all around me. Words were a passion of sorts with me. If they did not create my reality, they certainly gave it shape. I thought of the one word I did not want to enter into my personal collection, then said it quietly to myself: cancer. It had an inescapably fatal sound.

I immediately read myself the riot act for allowing my imagination to run away with me. My toughness had always seen me through hard times. I had the reputation of being a good person in a crisis. If this was to be a crisis, I would simply respond as others had grown to expect.

But I was still bowled over by what I'd just read. As if this worry had dislodged something from my past, I thought of the bookshelves of my childhood home. My father had been a writer and book collector. When a book arrived in the mail from New York or London, there was always great excitement. I loved the feel of those books in my hands. I loved the sound they made as I cracked open their spines in the precise way I had been taught by my father. I spent many happy hours carefully slicing open the uncut pages of first editions written by authors living between the time of Dante and Hemingway. At a very early age I was taught that books and writing were things to value and respect.

But as a child I had no thoughts of becoming a writer. I longed only to be an artist, as my mother was. Many of her sketches hung on the walls of our home. I could completely lose myself in trying to apply paint so deftly that there was no telling where one stroke began and the other ended.

I grew up in what is nowadays referred to as a dysfunctional family. I had recently looked up the word "dysfunctional" in *Roget's Thesaurus* and been unable to find it. But *dys* was there, with three cross-references: "abnormal," "bad," "difficult." My childhood was all of those things. I didn't think of it that way at the time—it was simply all I knew. It wasn't until my teen-age years that I allowed myself to consider how grim it was. I never doubted my parents' love, but my childhood was a confusing, frightening place to be, one that I tried to escape through whatever means available. My early years passed while I read, painted or fled to the nearby mountain. In school, I was often caught staring out the window or reading a book I had hidden in my desk.

The house had grown pitch-dark. I heard people with expectations coming up the front stairs and realized I must have fallen asleep. Full of energy and high spirits, my husband and daughters burst into the room. I cast a smile wide enough to take them all in at once and stood up to hug them, feeling beautifully drugged for a moment.

But then the word "cancer" came back to me. I felt numb, as though part of me had stayed asleep.

"You look tired," Peter said.

I yawned. "I dozed off. I'm not quite awake yet."

Jenny, my youngest, brought me a cup of tea and started telling me about her day. She loved to draw, and as she talked she doodled on the calendar I'd left beside me. I listened, lifting my cup with both hands and drinking as deeply as I could.

"Hey, what happens at two o'clock on Tuesday? You've only written in the time."

I was saved from having to answer by her older sister, Katherine, who stood in the middle of the stairway with a piece of plastic in her hand. "Who put *this* in the garbage?"

I let out a huge sigh. "Oh, I hope it wasn't me," I said, knowing I was the most likely culprit.

"Moz," she admonished, "don't you want to change?"

The name Moz was a combination of Mom and Roz, a blend suitable for a nineties mother-and-daughter relationship.

"I'm trying, Katherine. I swear to God I'm trying, but sometimes I think all those recklessly extravagant years of the fifties have ruined me forever."

She gave me a sad-eyed look. Katherine had found a cause in the environment and had formed a club at university known as SEA—Students for Environmental Action. Although I hoped she was involved only in peaceful action, I agreed with many of her views.

"Listen, I'm not all bad," I rationalized. "I do save lives."

The moment seemed appropriate to make my excuses. I walked up to the kitchen to find Peter unfazed by a wine cork that had self-destructed in the neck of a bottle.

"Would you like a glass if I can get to the wine?" he asked, smiling good-naturedly. He had changed into a casual blue shirt. I always loved to see him in blue. It brought out the colour of his eyes.

"Thanks, but I think I'll head upstairs to bed," I said. I would have liked a drink, but I was too tired and too aware of how vulnerable I'd be. I thought only briefly of telling him about the lump I'd found. Since my childhood, I'd been used to dealing with things on my own. And I didn't want to trouble him over something that might turn out all right.

I gave him a gentle kiss on the cheek.

He put down the bottle and wrapped his arms around me. "You've eaten, haven't you?" he asked.

"Yes," I lied.

I headed upstairs and stretched into the coolness of the sheets, naked. I listened to the sounds of the family: the dog's footsteps on the hardwood floor below me; my sixteen-year-old talking on the telephone to a friend; my nineteen-year-old, home from university for a study break, flipping through the pages of a textbook; Peter in the kitchen putting the finishing touches on some gourmet dinner for himself and the girls.

These were the rhythms of the house. Safely enclosed in their familiarity, I was reassured. I could live within the walls of this house forever, I thought.

I lay there drifting, almost asleep. Finally, I heard Peter come upstairs. Before getting into bed, he closed a window tight against the winter downpour. Snuggling against him, I made sure his hand did not go near my right breast.

2

THE DAYS ARE SHORT IN JANUARY. It was very dark when I got up at six o'clock the next morning and put on my uniform. I was grateful to be working that day; the demands of the job always allowed me to completely forget my own life. Only the patients were important. Decisions had to be right on target, actions fast and compassionate. Violence was routine, and I never knew what reserves I might have to call upon.

Our first response was to a head-on collision on the highway north of the ambulance station. It was my turn to attend to the patients, so my partner, Brian, drove. We sped down the road with the siren wailing and the emergency lights sweeping away the early-morning darkness. At the accident scene, the ambulance's wig-wags flashed on the wreckage of two vehicles scattered across the road. There was an eerie silence. A young female in a sports car was conscious but badly injured. There were two unconscious people in the other car. A quick assessment told me that we had three critical patients.

I reached for equipment. "Brian, do we have one or two other ambulances coming?"

"Two, Roz—one from the north and one from the south."

"The fire department for extrication?"

"They're on their way."

I could already hear more than one siren approaching in the distance. As the crews arrived, I triaged the patients according to injuries. I decided that Brian and I would transport the young woman as soon as she was freed from her car by the firefighters. We were the last ambulance to leave.

There was only a trickle of blood from the corner of the woman's mouth, but she showed signs of shock. I suspected she had internal injuries, and I also knew that her head had taken a blow. She was unable to answer my questions and kept saying over and over, "What happened … what happened?"

The closest trauma hospitals were a half-hour away. Brian put on the siren and we headed for the city. In the back of the ambulance, I worked on the patient and notified the hospital that we were coming in. Searching for hidden injuries, I cut away all her clothing, then covered her with several warm blankets. As we backed into Emergency, our patient was holding her own, but I was relieved to hand her over to the trauma team.

The day didn't let up. We responded to three more car accidents, a domestic dispute and several medical problems.

An elderly gentleman with a fractured hip saluted me, asking what the gold bars on my shoulders meant.

Brian told him, "They mean she's the boss."

"It means I get to do the paperwork." I smiled at them both.

Our last call of the day was the routine transfer of a patient from the hospital to the Cancer Agency for radiation treatment. Maggie had undergone a mastectomy several months before. Now she was in an advanced stage of the disease. She had bone metastasis, and recently the cancer had spread to her lungs. She needed to be kept on oxygen because she was constantly short of breath. The radiation treatments were simply for pain control. We had been transferring Maggie back and forth between the hospital and the Cancer Agency for several months, but I hadn't seen her for two weeks. Last time, she'd told me she had always been interested in becoming a paramedic and she was going to look into it. Then, startled by what she'd heard herself say, she'd attempted a smile, explaining that she talked about a future out of habit. I respected Maggie's courage, but today I had mixed feelings about seeing her.

There was no one at the nurses' station in the palliative care unit. While we waited, I flipped through a magazine. A glossy photo of bald women who looked like survivors of a concentration camp caught my attention. Each of the women had only one breast. The story's headline made it clear that I fit two of the major risk categories for breast cancer: I was a woman and I was aging. In the past thirty years, the article's opening lines said, little had been learned about a disease that had become the number-one killer of women between the ages of thirty-five and fifty-four. And few new treatments had been discovered during that time.

I heard a nurse coming down the hall. She seemed surprised to see us.

"We're here for Maggie," I explained.

"But we cancelled the transfer," she said. "Maggie passed away."

I felt both relieved and sad. At last, it was over for her. I wasn't shocked; I saw death all the time in my work. The body was designed to fail. But I was moved by the thought of someone who had lived so recently, and now ...

We headed back to the ambulance station. I was quieter than usual and grateful that Brian didn't comment on it. As soon as the night crew arrived, I changed quickly out of my uniform. I had only an hour before my art history class started.

By the time I reached the university, I was running through halls empty enough for a Sunday. I entered the lecture theatre just as the professor was telling the class, "This is not deformity, but an affair of shapes, the loveliness of possibility, where we can compare our symmetry with that portrayed by the artist."

I looked at the portrait by Picasso displayed on the overhead screen. Bold strokes of blue, white shadowing, a smudge of yellow for the lips. I stared hard at the woman's body: the overwhelming femininity, the impossible breasts.

More portraits of women flashed onto the screen. The professor described Picasso's cubist phase and the influence of collage on the art of film. My mind drifted until I was no longer listening. I could think only of the erotically charged paintings.

On the way back to Lions Bay, it started to snow. With the headlights angled low for the road and the wiper blades swishing back and forth, I drove slowly and carefully, enjoying the quietness and the lonely stretches of highway. But once I was in bed, I found myself awake and edgy.

I thought of the family photographs I had seen in Maggie's hospital room. When I'm working, I usually take the time to look at a patient's photos, partially out of curiosity but also as a way of starting conversation. One of the pictures of Maggie had been taken about ten years previously. I'd looked at her younger face for some indication that she sensed her life would end prematurely. But there was nothing. It had seemed a terrible warning to me at the time, I remembered now with some irony.

The snow had stopped. I listened to Peter's breathing. It was five o'clock and the moon had come clear. I still had a couple of hours before starting work, but I resigned myself to a lost night of sleep. I slipped my legs over the side of the bed and went down to my study. In the moonlight, the distant ocean appeared luminous. I turned on a lamp against what was left of the night.

Late the next afternoon, inside my office at the front of the Emergency building, I dreamily took in the winter landscape while I pressed a phone receiver against my ear. I had called the hospital's intensive care unit to get a report on the critical patient we'd transported the day before, and I'd been placed on hold. It had been a fairly quiet day. During a stop at a variety store, I'd browsed through a wall of magazines until I found a copy of the one I'd seen at the hospital. I flipped it open now to the article on breast cancer but couldn't concentrate. I switched the phone to my other ear and started a list of all the things I had to do. Then, feeling weary at the thought of the balancing act that would be required to accomplish everything, I scrunched up the list and threw it into the wastepaper basket. It started to unfold itself, growing larger and larger. I retrieved it and flattened it into the recycling bin.

"Okay," I said into the phone. "Thank you." The patient was still on the critical list, but her condition had improved remarkably.

As I heard the night crew coming up the stairs, I threw the magazine into my briefcase. Jeff poked his head in the door, smiled and looked at me questioningly.

"We took a woman into the hospital yesterday who was pretty badly injured," I said, just to say something. "She's going to make it."

"Good," he said. "Anything in particular you want us to do tonight?"

"If you wouldn't mind changing the main oxygen tank," I suggested. "It's down to a quarter."

"Consider it done. Anything else?"

I looked at him more closely. "Do you need extra points or something?"

He leaned his head sadly against the door frame. "I quit smoking. I need to be busy."

"Oh, if that's the case, feel free to wax the floors, clean the windows, strip the beds—"

"Enough," he shouted, climbing the remaining stairs two at a time.

"I'm going home," I yelled after him. "And no smoking when you change the oxygen tank. I don't want to see any missiles going past my windows."

"If you want to see some missiles, just turn on your television when you get home," he called back.

As I drove, I listened to the weatherman on the radio predict snow for the next day, followed by a warming trend and rain.

When I opened the front door, I saw Jenny sitting on the floor in front of the TV. The set was on, but the sound was turned down. Jenny wore faded overalls and a baseball cap turned back to front. For just an instant, it looked as if her head were on backwards. She was drawing.

"Hi, Mom," she said, concentrating on her work.

"Hi, darling." I took off my jacket and boots. I went over to her, removed her cap and pushed back the long brown hair that fell well below her shoulders. I gave her a kiss. "What's happening on television?"

"Oh, it's about the war," she complained.

I could hear Katherine upstairs roughhousing with Freyja. I looked at the pictures on the screen. The night sky was full of scarlet streaks, and on the ground people wearing gas masks ran for their lives between flaming buildings.

"Mom, is it still okay if I go on that ski trip?" Jenny asked.

"Hmm," I nodded, turning up the volume on the television.

A reporter's voice identified the city as Tel Aviv. "With the fear that one of the missiles might carry the promised poisonous gas, people are not taking any chances." The picture panned to the bright traceries in the sky. "Here you see a one-million-dollar Allied Patriot missile plunging from the sky to intercept an incoming Scud ... and there it is ... beautiful, a perfect strike for the anti-missile missile ... and there ... another one...." The film footage changed to Baghdad. Iraqis watched a Tomahawk missile skimming the Baghdad skyline.

I realized I had been holding my breath only when I began to breathe again. "My God," I said. "It's no wonder we get desensitized to the horrors of the world. There are just too many of them. Nothing amazes anyone any more."

Jenny glanced up at me for a moment, but she didn't say anything. When I walked upstairs I heard her turn the sound off again. I called out to Katherine and Freyja, who both charged down from the upstairs bedroom to see me.

"Has anyone around here eaten?" I asked.

"Freyja has eaten," Katherine said, giving me a hug. "I don't mind waiting for Dad to get home."

"Jenny, how about you?" I called down to her.

"I ate some stuff at Jen's," she replied, still not looking up from her work. I wondered briefly what kind of "stuff" it had been.

I decided to make some dinner for myself. Peter could feed the girls when he got home. Until I'd married I'd always thought that "marrying well" meant you had snagged someone with money or prestige. But I'd discovered that a low-maintenance male who loved to cook also fit into that category.

As I cleared a place for myself at the table, I picked up a sheet of paper. "What's this?" I asked.

Katherine looked at the drawing in my hand. "That's a bat house Dad wants to build."

"A bat house? Why does he want to build a bat house?"

"He likes bats," she answered, unperplexed. "He figures he can get rid of the insects in the summer if more bats are encouraged to live around here."

"Wonderful," I said, smiling to myself.

I never knew what might appear next. The previous summer, we'd had a problem with wasps. Peter constructed a frame so that he could suspend a fish head over a large pail of water. He set this contraption on top of an overturned barrel. The wasps flew up into the fish head, gorged themselves, fell into the water, and drowned.

As I started to eat dinner, Katherine sat down beside me, her beautiful mane of fair hair pulled loosely back and secured with an elastic band. She watched me as I ate. I glanced at her from time to time. She was by nature reflective, quiet and strong. Like her father, I thought.

"What have you been up to today?" I asked, through a mouthful of chicken.

"Just studying," she said in the faintest voice.

"That's what I should be doing," I said, chewing on a bone. Freyja had moved in and was monopolizing the floor on my side of the table, watching my every move.

Katherine eyed me for what seemed like a long time. "I don't know how you can stand eating meat."

"Old habits die hard," I said, wiping my face and feeling I'd fit right into the famous scene from *Tom Jones*. I pushed my chair away from the table, washed my hands and came back to sit down. Katherine held her chin in her hand, gazing out the window.

"When do you go back to university?" I asked.

"Tomorrow."

"How's the studying going?"

"Not so great. I'm not doing as well as last year. My heart's just not in it right now. But I'm sure that feeling will come and go like everything else."

"Very wise of you," I observed, and then added, "I don't work until tomorrow night. How about I drive you to the bus?"

"Thanks," she said, toying with a fork. "I'd like that."

Peter opened the front door just then, shook himself like a dog, and sent snow in every direction. "Brrrrrr," he said. "It's colder than the north side of a gravestone in winter."

Katherine's face lit up as she watched her father's display of the cold shivers.

"Hey, careful with my picture," Jenny shouted at him.

"I'm sorry," he apologized. "Did it get wet?"

"No, but it was close." She stood up to give him a hug.

I smiled, thinking that this was the longest Jenny ever got perturbed at anyone.

Peter played with Freyja for a minute or two and then called me downstairs. "I'm going to play you something very wonderful," he said, unwrapping a compact disk and slipping it into the CD player. "It's an Oscar Peterson recording that I thought you'd like."

I loosened his tie as he opened his arms. His cheek beside mine felt fresh and cool.

I listened to the gentle Latinish beginning. The music became very bluesy. It was joyous, it was sad, it whispered, it yelled. During a slow dazzling passage, I nodded at Peter approvingly.

"Yes," he said. "I couldn't pass it up."

I peered over his shoulder at pile upon pile of CDs. "Maybe we should put an addition on the house for the CDs you couldn't pass up."

"Good idea." He smiled, starting to dance with me.

Jenny grabbed her picture and fled downstairs, only half-complaining as she said with a grin, "Like, give me a break, you guys!"

As we turned around and around in front of the television, I shut my eyes against glimpses of a sky lit with streaking missiles and a street in flames.

3

THE SKY WAS A RARE BLUE on Tuesday. I went to my afternoon appointment with as much of a sense of business as usual as I was able to manage. I tried not to focus on the fact that Dr. Harris was a specialist in breast surgery. He's just a *specialist*, I reassured myself. The waiting room was disturbingly silent.

Half a dozen women sat in chairs, but there was no cozy female camaraderie, no smiles of support or understanding. The room was full of fear, I suddenly realized. It made me think of a Woody Allen line: It's not that I'm afraid to die—I just don't want to be there when it happens.

Eventually, a nurse took some information, then ushered me into the examination room. She asked me to remove my clothing down to the waist. I could hear the doctor talking to someone on the telephone in his office. His nurse had left a gown for me. As soon as I had changed, I browsed through a magazine. It was full of shots of the Gulf War. I tried to concentrate on how the photographer had imposed his art on the scenes, countering changes in subject matter and light with different lenses and speeds of film.

When the doctor opened the door, I was impressed immediately. He looked intelligent, fit and professional. I was comforted by his manner, too. He pulled up a stool and quietly asked me a series of questions.

"Any cancer in the family?"

"None that I'm aware of, but I don't know for sure … my father was adopted."

"Are your parents living?"

"No."

"How did they die?"

For the first time in my life, I considered the answer good news. "They took their own lives," I said as matter-of-factly as I could. For some obscure reason I always thought of it more as murder: my mother killed my father; my father killed my mother.

He raised one eyebrow and asked, "At the same time?"

"No."

He looked back at the form his nurse had started. "And your four older sisters … how is their health?"

I was happy to leave the old useless grief and pain behind. "My sisters are all well."

"Do you smoke?"

"Just a pipe. A bad habit I acquired from my husband. But I don't smoke all that often," I rationalized quickly.

"Well, let's have a look." He put down the chart and palpated my left breast, then my right.

"Hmm," he said as his practised fingers zeroed in on the mass. "It's a pretty good size, isn't it?" His eyes held mine until I looked away.

He completed his examination. "I don't think this is anything to worry about, but it certainly is quite a lump you have there. In all likelihood it's a cyst. I'm going to give you a little local freezing and use a needle to draw off the fluid. In a few minutes, you'll walk out of here without it. How does that sound?"

I felt an immediate stirring of hope. We bantered back and forth about how little was known about cysts and how no one was sure why some people were prone to getting them. He stuck a hypodermic needle into my breast, a painless procedure, and I watched for the fluid, like a genie, to appear in the syringe.

Then he pulled out the needle. The syringe was dry.

"Strange," he said, looking thoughtful. "Perhaps I missed it."

I gave him a fleeting smile. "You've got a pretty bad aim if you missed this one."

"It's happened before." He patted my arm lightly as if to reassure me. "If we're lucky, we'll have some microscopic tissue in this needle that the lab can examine."

I did not want the needle biopsy to fail. "Isn't it worth another try?"

"No, it's best not to disturb these things any more than we need to. I think we'll find we have some cells here that will tell us something."

I looked at the glass slide that he handled so meticulously. My fate rode on something I couldn't even see.

I put my clothing back on and followed him into his office.

"Have you had a mammogram recently?" he asked.

"No, the earliest appointment I could get is at the end of next week."

He picked up the telephone, and I listened as he talked to the mammography department. "Dr. Harris here. You have one of my patients, a Ms. Rosalind MacPhee, booked next week for a mammogram. I'd appreciate it if you could fit her in sooner than that."

There was a long pause before he continued. "You're that busy, are you?" He stared directly at me. "No, I'd like her fitted in tomorrow or the next day at the latest."

He waited patiently, tapping a pen on his desk. "Thank you," he said finally, and then he raised his eyebrows at me. "Can you go there now? It's just down the street."

I nodded.

He hung up and rang a buzzer to summon his nurse.

"Nancy, I'd like you to find an appointment time for Rosalind towards the end of this week. We should have the pathology report and the mammogram results by then."

I walked out into the busy street and stood there letting people bump into me. I looked up at the sky. The winter sun was slanting down between the tall buildings. It's not so bad, I told myself. Nothing is so bad if the sun is shining.

There wasn't much to having a mammogram. I waited until

my name was called and then I was shown to a small curtained cubicle. A technician handed me a gown. She asked me to leave it open at the front.

The lighting in the X-ray room was much brighter than in the waiting room. The technician asked me a few questions and then directed me to stand in front of a tall machine that looked like a pterodactyl. Each breast in turn was compressed between cool X-ray plates. I had to take a deep breath and hold it for a few seconds while the film was being exposed.

The technician asked me to wait while the pictures were checked to see if any views needed to be repeated. I watched the feet of other women beneath the curtain as they walked back and forth for their mammograms. Finally, I was told that I could get dressed and leave. The radiologist's report would be sent directly to my doctor.

Although I thought it was probably useless to ask, I decided to give it a try. "Can you see anything there?"

The technician smiled kindly. "There is some shadowing in the right breast," she said, "but only the radiologist can determine what it means."

I smiled back and nodded a thank you. It was more than I had expected her to say. I put my clothes back on and walked out through the waiting room with an uneasy sense of eyes watching me.

Driving home, I decided to visit my friend Deirdre, who was also a neighbour. Her house was a twenty-minute walk from mine, but in this mountain village everyone is considered a neighbour. I left the car in my driveway and walked over to see her.

As usual, she greeted me warmly. "What's happening?"

"Not much," I said. "How about you?" She poured us each a glass of wine. We settled side by side on stools at an island in her kitchen, discussing our children, the uncertain weather and our shock at the Gulf War.

"Did you see those incredible night shots from that bomber?" she asked.

I nodded. "Before they let go of the bombs, you could see the Euphrates and Tigris rivers."

"Poor old Mother Earth," she sighed. She assumed the dreamy expression she always wore when talking about any kind of motherhood.

Deirdre's father had died unexpectedly a month before. Although I had done my best to help her work through the loss, I suspected she was still struggling with a lot of unfinished business. I knew from experience that sudden death was especially difficult because it left so much unsaid, unexplored, unresolved. I also knew that Deirdre, at the age of sixteen, had lost her mother to breast cancer. I decided to keep my own news from her.

But she was intuitive about many things. She noticed the wooden beads I was wearing, gave them a tug and asked, "Hey, how come you're all dressed up?"

I smiled. "In the city doing errands," I told her.

The fact that we were so close amazed many of our friends because our styles as people were so different. They often joked about "how to explain Roz and Deirdre."

I was most comfortable in loose shirts and yesterday's jeans. For me, getting dressed up meant putting on a silk blouse, my wooden beads and a pair of tailored jeans. Deirdre had a flair for fashion and wore clothes well. Her hair was curly and loose and always made me think of the wind. The longish skirts she liked to wear flowed around her, giving an impression of unceasing movement. She had a soft look that I loved.

Deirdre's mission in life was her home and family. Her house, a subtle study of greys and whites, was tastefully and perfectly kept.

Domesticity didn't interest me at all. I expected the whole family to pull together to make our home livable. Only the study, with its piles of books, manuscripts and loose pages everywhere, was mine to deal with. And although I couldn't imagine anyone loving their family more than I did, I was manic in my need to be off on my own. I was always plotting ways to abandon my loved ones for days or weeks at a time.

Deirdre often joked that the biggest difference between us was that I wore glasses and she didn't. She said when she was quiet, people thought nothing was happening. But because I wore glasses, when I was quiet people assumed I was thinking. At some point I think we decided that, because our lives were so different, we offered each other a place to hide.

The two of us had become friends after she'd interviewed me following the publication of my second book of poetry; she wrote a review of my work for our local newspaper. She was curious and bright, and I loved to listen to her talk. Sometimes when I reached an impasse in my writing I'd tell her about it and she'd come up with a clever idea to put things back in motion. I enjoyed her company so much that I'd reorganize my day just to spend time with her. We'd both had small children when we met, and on warm days we'd pack them off to school, then throw my kayaks into the ocean and head for distant islands. We swore some kind of time warp occurred out on the water. Predictably, we'd be at a full run by the time we got back to the school to pick up the kids. Then, as now, we whiled away endless hours talking about ideas.

"What happens in a person's life is by choice," she said, twirling her wine glass.

I raised my glass to catch the winter sun through the window. I enjoyed arguing this point with her. "Maybe for some," I said, "but for most people in the world, life is a matter of survival. Take, for instance, the Kurdish refugees ..."

Deirdre's husband often arrived home to find his wife missing or me added to the scene. Today, he walked in as we were polishing off a bottle of Pinot Noir. He didn't seem to mind. He opened another bottle and poured a drink for himself, leaving the bottle within our reach.

"Trusting man." I grinned, pushing the bottle his way. I stood up to leave.

"Would you like a ride?" he asked.

"No, thanks," I said. "I feel like walking."

Happy, I set off for home. A short visit with Deirdre had made a difficult day agreeable. We had shared so much over the past dozen years that I expected our friendship would endure anything. But I was very glad we lived so close to one another. I had a history of losing interest in anyone who didn't constantly stay in touch. Deirdre often gave me a hard time about this. She said my reaction to separation was not normal. I tended to live very much in the present—if people were not there at that moment, they ceased to exist.

A year or two after Deirdre and I met, a greatly loved friend of mine moved to Sweden. Deirdre was very understanding and supportive. But she couldn't resist bringing a little humour into my struggle. On one occasion she screwed up her face to look like an insect, brought her head very close to mine and said, "So what happens to you ... do you lose your antennae?"

Shortly after that, Deirdre too moved away from Lions Bay, so she was able to test my reaction for herself. At first, I felt a strange dazedness I could liken only to the aura that warns of an epileptic seizure. Still, I rallied: hosting a good-bye party;

helping her clean, pack, unpack and paint; providing meals and hugs. After she'd moved, I put in a real effort to keep the connection. But we soon saw less and less of each other. Two years later, she and her family moved back to Lions Bay— "because of people," she said. Within hours, we were back into our old habit of seeing each other or talking almost daily.

For the next few days I went to work and studied whenever I could. I had a term paper due, but even though I opened books, I barely glanced at the words. I sat at my desk and watched my pipe smoke drift aimlessly towards the skylight. I listened to the radio without taking anything in. I tried to think basics: hot and cold water, bills to be paid, the dog to be walked. But unsettling thoughts were always in the back of my head. I wandered through the house untangling the vacuum, watering plants and moving books from one room to another. It was more and more difficult to write. Many of my poems were short and fragmented. *Believing the island out here is a moment of sun ... our hard bed of light, stripped by the salt wind that fumbles at my clothes ... the sea in your eyes has the blue feel of love.*

One cold afternoon as I arrived home from shopping, Peter pulled into the driveway behind me.

"You're home early," I said, loading his arms with groceries.

"Unfortunately, it's to pack. I have to be at the airport in a couple of hours."

"How long will you be away?"

"The better part of a week." He was full of apologies, since the next day was my birthday. "Where's Jenny?" he asked.

"Skiing until the end of the week. It's some kind of professional development break for teachers."

"I thought she'd be back," he said, dumping the bags down on the kitchen counter.

"Not to worry," I reassured him. "I'm old enough not only to be alone on my birthday but to enjoy it." We talked while I put groceries away. Although I couldn't recall ever wanting him to be at home as much as I did just now, I sent him off with a packed suitcase and a smile.

I chatted on the phone with Deirdre while I cooked myself some dinner, the pots and pans miraculously arranging themselves on the stove. After I'd eaten, I roamed the house, picking up the detritus of a busy week. It wasn't true that I was old enough to enjoy being alone on my birthday. The day before my eleventh birthday, my father had taken his life, and my childhood had taken one of its many calamitous turns. Although my mother didn't wander off into a snowdrift with a bottle of gin until much later, she locked herself in a bedroom and was lost to me in any tangible fashion from that night on. For a long time I had hoped my mother would suddenly materialize out of the shadows of my new life, but it was not to be. Looking back on those years, I saw them as a series of dissolves, utterly distanced.

I wondered briefly what a woman alone should do on the eve of her birthday. Ignore it, I decided. At all costs, not think of it as possibly her last. I knocked off a few quick sit-ups. Then I decided to catch up on my assignments. I poured myself a drink, carried my books downstairs, put on some music, stretched out on the sofa, and dove into reading about the fearless Picasso, who would actually allow people to watch him paint.

Finally, I went to bed. It was after midnight. I lay awake for a long time in the darkness.

I woke to Freyja's barking. Glancing at my watch in the dark, I saw that it was only five o'clock. I heard the muffled rise and fall of voices, and then a stampede of sound coming up the stairs, pots and pans being banged together, women singing: "When you're forty-five and still alive, from friends like us there's no place to hide."

Faces surrounded my bed. Deirdre took my hand and wrapped my fingers around a glass of Kahlúa and milk. My friend Pat was making some kind of speech. I was still dozy, but I caught the gist of her words. "Well, my sweet, we heard your man was out of town, so we'll just have to do."

Pat started to put baskets on the floor. "We've brought breakfast and lunch and dinner—we're here for the day whether you are or not."

A woman I'd never seen before put out her hand to shake mine. "Hi, I'm Jacki."

I laughed. "Hi, I'm Rosalind. Do I know you?"

"You do now," she said. "I'm from Montreal, but I'm here visiting one of your crazy friends. I'm Jennifer's sister. When Jennifer asked if I wanted to have some fun, I thought, Sure— I've never started a party at five in the morning before."

I was wishing I had worn something respectable to bed. Instead, I had on an old pyjama top appliquéd with a partly eaten apple. Pat threw me my ragged housecoat and suggested I make myself decent.

"What I'd like is a quick shower," I said. "Obviously you can make yourselves at home for that long."

Towelling off, I listened to all the familiar voices. I'd known many of these friends even longer than Deirdre. They were housewives, nurses, teachers and flight attendants. There was a musician, a potter, a real estate agent and even a fitness expert. I overheard the stranger named Jacki tell Brenda, our local counselling psychologist, that she should run for mayor. I smiled: Jacki had fit right in. I looked at my watch again. It was 5:20, and a party was in full swing.

When I came down to join them, Deirdre was amusing the group. She had put on a pair of my glasses and placed a pipe in her mouth. The entertainment continued until Marilyn approached me bearing a candlelit cake. Everyone started to sing. I leaned into the heat and brightness to blow.

"So, are you a little surprised?" Marcia asked.

I nodded my head, laughing. "Did Peter know about this?"

"Yes, but he swore not to tell. We wanted to make sure you were going to be home and not hauling bodies off the highway." Pat held out her arms and gave me an engulfing hug. "Happy birthday, old thing."

My friendship with Pat had had what I'd always referred to as a no-shit beginning. Eight years earlier, a rock slide had buried her teen-aged sons Tom and David along with her home and belongings. Pat's family had been asleep when the slide hit. In the early-morning light of the next day, I had watched her, along with her husband and their three daughters, wait quietly while the bodies of the two boys were dug out of the mud.

A few days later I was asked by our local council if I would organize work parties to go through the rubble of several houses that had been destroyed. The village clerk explained to me, "It needs a woman's touch, Rosalind, someone who can understand what it means to see a stranger with a chain saw cutting through your grand piano after it's been buried by mud."

My work party spent a month trying to salvage things that might be of importance: diaries, silverware, cookbooks, photographs. Sometimes it meant standing in front of heavy equipment defying the operator to run you down while you scooped a wedding ring or retrieved a family portrait. On one of the demolition days, Pat came by to say she was concerned about how hard I was working. She invited me to have a drink with her in the accommodation that had been found for her family. When we had polished off one bottle of wine, we uncorked the next. We drank until we were satisfied with the excavation, the rainy weather, and even the lives we had led up until then.

"Rosalind," Pat called now. "This is unbelievable. I was just trying to figure out why I recognized Jacki." Pat swept her hand dramatically through the air as if introducing Jacki on stage: "She used to be lead singer with the Bells—a Montreal group. I have some of her records," Pat said, putting her arm around Jacki. "Rosalind, you salvaged them from the slide."

"Records survived that slide?" Jacki asked.

"We kept the records in the dining room," Pat said. "Not much happened to the dining room. It just got moved."

Pat was easy to love for her humour and indomitable spirit. A big woman in every sense of the word, she was excessive in warmth, caring and generosity. Ever since one of my previous birthdays, when she had commandeered the Vancouver Chamber Choir to sing "Happy Birthday" to me from a pay phone, I had held her in awe.

She was also the intelligence operative in our network of friends—all information passed through Pat. We relied on her to be our social convener. When the "Lions Bay Luncheon Ladies" got together, Pat always told her husband that she was going to a "board meeting." At this moment, she was waving her camera in the air and saying expansively, "Beauties ... beauties ... I told Mike I was going to a board meeting. He didn't believe me." With an expression of mock-surprise, she added, "I can't imagine why. So I want proof."

She took a number of pictures of us all smiling out at the world. My smile was as big as everyone else's. I wondered if, when these pictures were developed, others would be able to tell from the look on my face that I feared what was coming.

4

IT WAS A FINE MORNING. It seemed much like any other fine morning until the doctor handed me two pieces of paper. The pathology report stated that the mass in my breast had atypical cells that were "worrisome." How strange to find the word "worrisome" in a medical report, I thought. Immediate removal of the mass was recommended. The mammogram report, one sentence long, told me that my mammogram was normal and that I should repeat the test in a year. I gazed at the papers as if they were written in code.

I only half-heard the words coming out of my mouth. "If there's a tumour there, why doesn't the mammogram show it?"

"Sometimes a tumour is made up of the same cells as the rest of the breast tissue—there isn't enough contrast for the tumour to show on the X-ray." When I didn't respond, Dr. Harris added, "I've been burnt by mammograms before. You know and I know there is something there." I handed the reports back to him.

He held the flimsy pieces of paper in the air. "I'm recommending that we do an incisional biopsy as day surgery at the hospital. Because this will be very much on your mind, I think it would be wise to do so as soon as possible."

"Is there anything else we should do before this biopsy?"

"I could send you for an ultrasound—that would tell us if it's a cyst. But because of the atypical cells, I would recommend we book a time in the hospital. Then you'll know exactly what you're dealing with."

"And if it is cancer …?"

"God forbid. I'll cut around the tumour—nothing beyond that. We'll do a frozen section while you are under the anaesthetic."

"A frozen section?"

"Yes. A thin slice of the lump is examined by a pathologist during the surgery. That way we'll know whether or not it is cancer. If it is, the tumour gets sent to the lab so we know what kind of cancer we are dealing with. And then you and I get together and talk … make our decisions from there."

I had anticipated that he would say, "If it's cancer, don't worry—there's still lots we can do. Breast cancer can be cured." Instead, he had used the expression "God forbid." I wondered if he knew what those two little words meant to me. They told me that if the cells were malignant—situation disaster.

I felt the palms of my hands grow moist. "How long will it take to get into the hospital?"

"Probably only a week or two. The hospital is very understanding about these kinds of biopsies."

I nodded but remained silent.

"If you would like to discuss this with your husband, or friends, you could call me with your decision. I wouldn't leave it too long—it's going to weigh on your mind."

"That's not necessary," I said. "You can go ahead and book the surgery." He looked me over for a moment, then said his nurse would call me as soon as they had a date.

I walked outside and stood on the sidewalk, dazed. I looked up and watched the slow passage of a jet cut the sky like a knife through paper.

As I drove home, I wondered if I should get a second opinion about my diagnosis. Dr. Harris was certainly amenable to the idea of my talking to other surgeons. I knew that the Cancer

Agency was one of the best hospitals in the country. I knew I would recommend it to anyone else. But I also believed it was only wishful thinking that another doctor might obtain different results from a needle biopsy.

Dr. Harris was providing me with the information I felt I needed; so far, he'd been instrumental in making the tests and procedures happen immediately; he'd assured me there would be ongoing communications between us before any decisions were made. Furthermore, I knew his reputation—people survived surgery under his care.

But what especially drew me towards him was that he made me feel my life mattered to him. When he looked at me, his eyes seemed to say, "I want you to get through this." I liked him. And I believed he had a sense of the individual catastrophe of cancer.

By the time I got home there was a message on my answering machine from Dr. Harris's nurse. "Ms. MacPhee, the hospital can schedule you for the biopsy tomorrow morning. Please call us right away if this would be convenient."

Convenient? A problematic word. I knew I could get off work, but Peter was out of town, Katherine was back at university and Jenny was still away skiing. I might be able to drive myself to the surgery; however, I'd never get myself home after a general anaesthetic. Wanting it all over with as soon as possible, I confirmed I would be there in the morning and agreed not to eat or drink anything after midnight.

I selected a good bottle of Châteauneuf-du-Pape and walked over to Deirdre's. I pried her away from the preparations for the family dinner by uncorking the wine and pouring it into two tall glasses. When she noticed the label, she said, "Hey, what are we celebrating?" Her eyes flashed with something—regret or hope, I couldn't tell. She held her breath and said quickly,

"Please tell me it isn't something I'm supposed to have remembered."

I took a sip of the wonderful wine. Deirdre had earned a reputation for being forgetful. I often needled her that it was difficult to build a friendship with someone who had no memory. She teased back that it was hard to stay friends with someone who decided you had ceased to exist whenever you disappeared from sight.

"Actually, I have to go into the hospital for day surgery tomorrow." I impressed myself with the nothing-much-has-happened tone of my voice. "Everyone's away at my place … would you have time to play chauffeur?"

Deirdre stood in the middle of the kitchen, the knife she held suspended in the air. "Of course. Surgery for what?"

"I have a lump in my right breast. It needs to become history."

"Since when?" she asked, absentmindedly cutting the air.

I'd never known Deirdre to be so short of words. "I've had it for a while. I thought it would disappear, but it hasn't. I've had a needle biopsy … there are some 'worrisome' cells."

Deirdre hadn't taken her eyes off me. I put my hand on top of hers. "Deirdre, will you stop waving the knife around? Knives make me a little nervous right now."

She put it down on the counter and gave me a long hug. "Roz, I don't need this right now," she said quietly.

Neither do I, I thought, neither do I.

It was a clear, cold night as I walked home. The house had never seemed so empty. My last night as a goddess and there was no one in my bed to hold my perfect body.

Deirdre picked me up early the next morning. She gave me an affectionate punch on the arm and made a joke about the extent to which I'd go just to sneak a new experience into a day. I noticed her eyes were watery, inquiring.

"No big deal," I said, smiling widely.

We spoke little on the way to the hospital. We entered through a side entrance, trying to avoid any nurses I might know and the inevitable question: "Roz, what are you doing here?" Halls that I walked through regularly closed in on me.

I looked at Deirdre, knowing that memories of the recent long hours in hospital with her father must be flooding back to her. She glanced around as if assassins were shadowing her.

"Listen, off you go ... I'll ask them to call you when I'm ready to leave."

She gave me a supportive hug. "I just know you're going to be okay," she said. "I just know it." And with a gentle pat on my cheek, she was gone.

Her words didn't comfort me. Deirdre saw life the way she wanted it to be. She had the ability to see potential in something half-finished, or not yet started—a highly desirable quality for a friend of a writer. But by her own admission, there was almost a fairy-tale dimension to how she viewed the world. We had often joked about her "rose-coloured glasses." It made me sad to realize that what was happening to me didn't fit into the kind of fairy tale she liked.

A clerk asked me questions, filling in the blank spaces on my admittance form.

"And what is your profession?"

I hesitated for a minute. Housewife? Poet? "Paramedic."

"Oh, I thought I recognized you." She smiled.

She indicated where I should sign to consent to surgery and absolve the hospital of responsibility for any valuables I might have brought in with me. "My life," I smiled at her. "I have only brought in my life."

The clerk placed some surgical tape around my wedding ring and handed me a green gown, long cotton leg-warmers and a hair net. As soon as my clothing was locked away, I walked out into a large room with two rows of beds. Many of the beds were already filled. Some patients were clearly waiting for surgery, leafing through magazines or looking about the room with restless eyes. Others appeared to be struggling to surface from anaesthetics.

A nurse took my temperature, pulse and blood pressure and explained that there was going to be a long delay. "There have been some unexpected emergencies," she explained. "All the scheduled surgeries have been pushed along."

She wrote down some information on the chart at the end of my bed and added, "I know waiting for surgery isn't very nice, but just try not to think about it."

You've got to be kidding, I thought, annoyed. I glanced at the big round clock on the wall. It was nine o'clock.

I made an effort to browse through a few magazines, and then I heard "Code Blue" repeated several times on the hospital announcement system. I knew someone wasn't making it through surgery. I put the magazines away and lay motionless, with my eyes closed. I thought of the manuscripts I'd figured I had years to finish. I tried to think of nothing. Nothing at all.

It was three o'clock in the afternoon before it was my turn. I hadn't had anything to eat or drink since the evening before; I felt very thirsty and had developed a splitting headache. At least the anaesthetic would take care of that.

Finally, they wheeled me into the operating room. A nurse slid a narrow board out from the left side of the operating table and secured my arm to it. A man who introduced himself as my anaesthetist lightly patted my veins, looking for the best insertion site.

The anaesthetist wrapped a tourniquet around my forearm and asked me to clench and then open my fist. This was a strategy to increase the blood flow to the area and make needle penetration easier. I sensed he was having difficulty finding a good vein. From my own experience in starting IVs, I recognized all the signs. It had been so long since I'd had anything to drink that my veins were not as spongy and full as we both would have liked.

He asked me to take a deep breath as he entered the skin. I watched for a flashback of blood indicating that the catheter was in the vein, but there was none.

"That's too bad," he said. "We like to use those large veins since we can get lots of fluid into them, and they pose less risk of perforation."

He chose another site higher up on the inside of my arm, cleansed the area and continued to explain, "We don't like to use these veins because sometimes people under anaesthetic have seizures and their arms jerk back on the needle."

By this time, the nurses were also watching for the flashback of blood. Still, it did not appear.

"Not to worry," he commented, looking very distressed. "We can always use these little veins here. We don't if we can help it, though, because the veins are so small we can't get much fluid into you if you start to hemorrhage."

I didn't want to hear it—any of it. What had happened to the concept of reassuring the patient?

A surgeon entered the operating room as yet another attempt was being made to start the intravenous. He wore a face mask, and until he talked to me I wasn't sure it was Dr. Harris.

"Trouble with the IV?" he asked.

The anaesthetist didn't answer, but as he released the tourniquet, I knew that this time he'd finally gotten a line—in a small vein. I said quietly, "I feel like a voodoo doll. I'd better pray I don't hemorrhage."

The last thing I heard before going under was my doctor saying, "You should have given the needle to Rosalind. She could probably have started her own IV without any problem."

When I came to, Dr. Harris was standing beside me in the recovery room. I was aware of small pools of fluid on my eyelids. As some of it ran down into my hair, I knew it had to be tears. I felt very sad. Somewhere way back in my brain, words were tumbling around in the darkness: "Doesn't look good ... doesn't look ... good."

Dr. Harris asked me how I felt. I told him I was very sore. He promised to order another shot of morphine for me. Despite the effects of the anaesthetic and the deep pull of sleep, the silence was unbearable.

Finally I asked, "What was it?"

He answered quietly, "It is cancer."

Another moment, or several moments, went by. Then I asked, "Where do we go from here?"

I was in a bubble. I saw his mouth moving and I was aware of a flow of words, but I was unable to process most of the information. He might as well have been speaking a different language. The diagnosis of breast cancer had taken over. I knew he'd said I would have to wait for the pathology report before I'd know if the cancer had spread beyond the tissue he'd removed. I knew I was to make an appointment to see him towards the end of the week.

I spent another hour or two in the recovery room mercifully asleep. And then I woke fighting nausea. I asked a nurse for a shot of Gravol. I was surprised that my stomach was so upset—I had previously tolerated morphine well. Then I remembered going under the anaesthetic and decided that no further explanation was necessary. It may have been a miracle that I woke up at all.

By the time my bed was pushed from the recovery room back to the day surgery ward, I was spending more time awake than asleep. The clock on the wall told me it was eight o'clock in the evening. There were only two other patients left in the ward.

The nurse was one I hadn't seen before. I realized there must have been a shift change. She was efficiently pleasant, taking a set of vitals before offering me a cup of tea.

"Are you hungry?" she asked, handing me a small tray.

Surprisingly, I was. I wolfed down two soggy sandwiches made from some mystery meat. The nausea got worse. I reached for a bowl.

Although the morphine was wearing off, I was more aware of soreness than pain. My hand gently explored the unfamiliar dressings that covered my right breast.

"Your friend is here to take you home." The nurse was annoyingly cheerful, handing me my clothing. "Are you feeling well enough?"

I knew that by this time I was the last patient there. "Let's give it a try," I said.

"Don't try to stand up yet. You'll find you're too woozy to do that."

While I lay on the bed, she helped me pull on my blue jeans. I was almost defeated by the challenge. It seemed there were leg openings everywhere, an endless series of blue tunnels that kept disappearing as soon as I thought I had found the right one.

I was hit by another wave of nausea. I didn't move until it passed. Under normal circumstances I knew I would fight the prospect of being pushed in a wheelchair. But not tonight. I rode submissively out to Deirdre in the waiting room.

"Hi," she said. She had a warm smile that made me feel safe.

"Hi."

"How are you doing?"

"Fine."

"Did she behave herself?" Deirdre asked. "She quite often doesn't, you know."

The nurse smiled and responded lightly, "She's had a bit of a rough time."

As I was loaded into my friend's small car, it occurred to me that sooner or later I was going to have to get out again. It was a daunting thought. Deirdre leaned over me to do up my seat belt, but I placed my hand gently on hers. "Please, don't bother. I'm a little sore."

We drove along the busy city streets in silence. When we hit the highway, she asked, "You okay?"

"It's cancer," I said.

She didn't say anything, but I was aware that she had turned her head to look at me. I leaned back and closed my eyes for a moment, concentrating on controlling my queasy stomach. We drove the rest of the way home in darkness and silence, each staring out our separate sides of the windshield.

As Deirdre pulled into my driveway, I realized I hadn't thought to leave the outdoor lights on. It was a long walk to the house, and then I would have to climb all those stairs to the front door.

Deirdre was grinning. "You don't like to make things easy for yourself, do you?"

"Sorry," I said, pushing open the car door.

"No, don't you move. I'm going to take you home with me. You can crash on the living room sofa."

"No thanks, Deirdre. Please, I'll be fine at home."

"Listen, my family will walk around you like you're not even there. You can play invisible."

"Deirdre, no. I'm fine at home—I *want* to be at home."

She opened her car door and sighed. "I guess I should have known you'd be this stubborn. Okay, you stay put."

I didn't argue. I listened to the sounds of a woman stumbling her way through the impermeable blackness of the forest. I heard the sound of Freyja's bark and knew Deirdre must have made it to the stairs.

As soon as the lights were on, she came back and helped me into bed. I asked her to feed Freyja but I declined her offer to stay with me for the night. I wanted only to stop all motion. I fell fast asleep, fully dressed.

When I awoke, the sky was a manageable blue. I felt strangely alert and rested, grateful for the long, deep sleep. I could remember Deirdre helping me onto the bed and nothing after that.

I ate a large breakfast and talked to Freyja as she prowled from one room to another, probably looking for the rest of her people. She was confident that this was her doghouse, particularly the dining room and kitchen. After breakfast I took her out for her regular morning walk. She loped along, stopping briefly to sniff the bushes or grass here and there. We always referred to this behaviour as "reading the daily news"—determining which dogs had recently been out and what they had been doing. She took off, chasing something real or imaginary, but soon caught up with me again. When we got home there was a note tucked under the front door: "I come over at the crack of dawn with coffee and homemade muffins and you don't answer the door. I let myself in because I figure you've fallen down the stairs and broken your neck or collapsed somewhere but I can't find you. Happily, I can't find Freyja either. I can only assume that some miraculous recovery has happened and you're both out walking. Please call. Love, Deirdre."

I walked over to see her.

"Look at you—all bright-eyed. I thought you'd be right out of it today."

"Actually, I feel pretty good. A little weak, but nothing that's going to get in the way."

She warmed her muffins in the microwave and I ate three of them, as if I'd had no breakfast at all. Then she drove me home. We didn't mention the word "cancer" once.

5

FOR THE NEXT TWO DAYS I worked night shifts, six at night until eight in the morning. Every time I lifted a patient I'd look down to see if my white shirt had turned red. I was uncomfortable enough to have difficulty sleeping during the daytime, and by the end of the two shifts I was exhausted. I flicked through endless TV channels and thought about university work I should be doing. No matter what I did, I was preoccupied with receiving the results of the lab tests that afternoon.

The phone rang. It was Duncan, my family doctor, asking me to come in for a talk with him after I saw Dr. Harris. We agreed on five o'clock.

I hung up. Not a good sign.

I went back to the television and heard a man's voice say quietly, "Advances in treatment have achieved only modest increases in survival rates. Only one in three of the women diagnosed with this disease will die of something else." I felt the hair on my head stand on end. I turned up the volume. There was film footage of a stadium full of women. They were all shouting and cheering. Then the shot flicked from colour to a still frame in black and white. There was no sound until the narrator's voice was heard again. "In Canada, this is the number of women who will die of breast cancer this year."

The rest of the documentary showed technicians working on computer simulations of rapidly multiplying cancer cells. But I didn't absorb anything else. I just lay on the sofa in a stupor, trying to get used to the idea that I was one of the statistics.

Eventually, it was time for my first appointment. I sat in Dr. Harris's waiting room staring at a wall of pamphlets: "Learning to Live with Cancer," "After Surgery," "Questions and Answers about Breast Cancer." Pamphlets that until now had been relevant only to other people, not to me.

I studied the other patients as discreetly as I could. A nurse spoke in whispers to one woman, who left the office in tears. Although no one made a move to comfort her, all eyes followed. She had left her jacket slumped headless in the chair beside me.

The nurse called out my name. I took a deep breath and got to my feet. Slowly, I said to myself, slowly.

The cancer had extended beyond the tissue removed. Dr. Harris set up appointments for scans, X-rays and a multitude of other tests. I heard percentages for survival rates: two, five, ten years. Was he talking to me? Two years seemed like next week. Mastectomy. Lumpectomy. With or without radiation. With or without the dreaded chemotherapy. He recommended a mastectomy, warning that the surgery would have the same impact as an amputation.

"I'm happy to refer you to the Cancer Agency—there are three doctors there who deal with nothing but breast cancer," he offered. "It's the best place to get a second opinion and more information. You have time to make the right decisions for yourself—that's very important. But most women want to have it looked after as soon as possible. Talk to your family and let me know when you've made your decision."

I left his office, my mind blank. I should have brought a friend or a tape recorder with me, I thought. It was only itinerary that moved me from one doctor's office to the next.

I had known Duncan since I was pregnant with Jenny. I knew he was supportive, a good listener, but I'd never been a person to talk much when it came to anything about myself. Today, I was even more reserved. At first, he received a lot of one- or two-word answers to his questions.

"How is the family handling it?" he asked.

"I haven't told them."

He shifted his weight in his chair. "Don't you think they should know?"

"I haven't wanted to worry them, at least not until I knew if there was something to worry about."

"Would you like me to speak to Peter?"

"I don't think—" my voice broke a little, whether from tiredness or the approach of tears, I wasn't sure. I felt as if I'd stumbled on uneven ground. "I can't do this to them."

He argued gently. "But they need to know. You can't do this on your own. You need more surgery, and that will probably be followed by treatments of one sort or another."

"I know … I will tell them," I said, and paused only long enough to feel the difficulty of the next question. "What do you think my chances of survival are?"

"We won't know that until after the next surgery."

"I guess I should probably have a living will made up."

"A good idea," he said. "It can help us to make decisions down the road."

His reply startled me. I had expected him to say, "Not to worry. You're going to be just fine—a living will is not necessary." More and more, I sensed that the process of this disease was not just physical but also emotional and psychological— an assaultive process that built until it created a sustained terror. This conversation was not about some patient in the back of an ambulance. This was me.

We both sat silently. Duncan studied my face. I looked away, then back.

"I need two years," I told him. "I need you to help me make decisions that will keep me around that long. Katherine can fly on her own, but Jenny needs a mother for two more years." I thought briefly of how Deirdre had lost her mother to breast cancer, then took a deep breath and added, "Sixteen is a hell of a time to lose a parent."

"Your chances of a good recovery are excellent," he reassured me. "If the woman who came in to see me this morning asked for two years I'd say her chances were very slim. She knew she had a lump a year ago and did nothing about it."

I realized I wasn't interested in the other woman. I wanted to go home. I stood up to leave. "Thank you," I said—for what, I wasn't sure.

He stood too. "Roz, you're going to have good days and you're going to have bad days … that's just the way it works. If you ever want to talk, let the receptionist know and she'll fit you in."

At home there was a message from Deirdre on my answering machine. When I called her back, she answered immediately. I could tell she was on her cordless phone. She sounded far away. And tired.

"Hi, it's me."

"How did it go?"

"I have to decide whether or not to have a mastectomy."

There was a long pause. I could hear the sounds of her family in the background. Music playing. It got louder for a moment as if someone had turned the wrong dial. She said, "I'm coming over."

"Actually, I'm done in, Deirdre. I kind of feel the way I do after a really bad day at work. Right now I just want some down time and some sleep."

"Are you sure?"

"Yes. Everything is under control." There was another pause. "What's all that noise?" I asked. "It sounds like Niagara Falls."

"Blender," she said. "Sorry." The noise stopped. "If you change your mind, call me. Promise me that."

"Yes, I promise."

"I'll talk to you tomorrow, then."

"If I'm still alive." She was silent. "Just kidding," I said.

After I hung up, I smiled a little at the idea that I was in control. I knew my ordeal had hardly started. I had a life-threatening disease, and I hadn't had enough of touching, of kisses, of sunshine, of mountains, of wonder, of laughter. I wanted it all.

The doctors' words kept tumbling around in my head. Dr. Harris's suggestion that I see the doctors at the Cancer Agency seemed reasonable. I had always been impressed by the surprisingly good spirits and helpfulness of its medical staff. But I was used to being at the Cancer Agency as a paramedic and I dreaded the thought of being there as a patient. No longer that pathetic relief—them, not me.

I sat in front of the television, flicking indecisively through the channels. I was afraid of what I might come across. But there were only new pictures released from Kuwait. I stared at a dark and surrealistic landscape, listening to dynamited well-heads roar like jet engines.

A scientist painted a picture of black beaches covered with dead fish, dead birds and other shapes so encrusted they couldn't be identified. He said the pall of smoke that filled the sky was loaded with carcinogens. "The chemicals from the fires will enter the milk of sheep, goats, camels and cattle through respiration and feed." I let my fingers pass lightly over my dressings, feeling for blood.

I flicked to another station. A four-star general talked excitedly about how a "smart" bomb could be custom-built for a special job within a matter of hours. Cameras were placed inside some of these bombs so that the viewer could approach a target just as if he or she were the bomb itself. An aerial view from a strike aircraft was shown. The pilot held the crosshairs squarely on a Baghdad rooftop. As the bomb honed in on its target, the bomb and I chased Iraqis through doors and down air shafts.

I turned off the television and headed upstairs. I climbed into bed, staring out at the cloudless night sky. The moon was the colour of aluminum. Where, I wondered, was the smart bomb for breast cancer?

At a time in my life when I had believed that my dreams could take me anywhere, I now feared I was as old as I would ever be. Would I be one of those who were diagnosed one day and dead a few weeks later? Or would there be time for family and friends, time for unfinished business, time to live before my own foregone conclusion—my death?

What I kept coming back to was: This is not how I am supposed to die. Violence had been part of my childhood and was now routinized by my job. Terror was on the highways and the streets. I had always thought an external force would bring about my end—not betrayal by my own body.

Freyja had traipsed upstairs, and she stood beside me hoping for an invitation onto the bed. I patted the quilt and she climbed up, turning in several slow circles before settling down against me.

I woke to the sound of the telephone ringing. In a daze, I answered, "Hello?"

Deirdre asked brightly, "And how are we this morning?"

"Actually, I didn't sleep very well," I admitted.

"I can't imagine why," she teased. Then she asked in a serious tone, "Are you in pain?"

"No, it's not bad. Really, it's more sore than painful. I just couldn't find the off switch for my brain last night. It was close to five by the time I fell asleep."

"And I've just woken you—"

"Not a problem. I need to be up anyway."

"What time does Peter get home?"

I glanced at my watch. "Any time now." I looked down at my dressings. "I'd better have a shower of some sort and make myself presentable."

"Good luck. I'm thinking of you."

"Thanks, Deirdre. I'll call you later."

Pulling on my blue jeans reminded me that the sun was shining. A perfect winter day. I had just finished tying my running shoes when Peter arrived. His tie was pulled loose from his collar and he looked tired. As always, Freyja managed to get to him before I did, so I had to wait my turn.

We held each other for a long time. Comfort and relief flooded through me.

"How are you?" he asked.

"Fine. And you?"

"I'm tired, and awfully glad to be home."

We sat and drank a cup of coffee, talking over his week. He'd been off in distant places attempting to solve acoustical problems that no one else could solve.

"What's new around here?" he asked, blowing one ropy circle of his pipe smoke through another.

"Jenny comes back from skiing today. It's been pretty quiet without her."

"I'm envious," he said. "A quiet week sounds wonderful."

I stretched. "It's a beautiful day. Will you walk down to the water with me?"

"Sure," he said, calling Freyja to join us.

It was one of those winter days that is so warm it startles you. We walked to the ocean holding hands and enjoying the fresh Pacific air. Freyja was in such an investigative mood that it took us close to an hour to cover what normally takes twenty minutes. When we reached the water, Peter stopped to throw some sticks for the dog.

I headed out onto the beach to sit on a big rock. The light reflected off the water. A raft of scoters lifted, flying low, departing. I watched the waves. I knew there were many people who thought of me as always being on top of a wave.

A cedar tree on the cliff above me was making soft, whispery sounds. I looked up past the branches into the blue as though memorizing the sky. White gulls were held by the wind like three crescent moons. Peter walked towards me. He said I looked like something that had been abandoned on the beach, waiting for the tide to come back and carry it away.

I smiled and patted the space beside me. "Here, come and share my rock."

I was reassured by the warmth of his familiar body next to mine. We sat in silence, as we often did.

"You seem preoccupied," he said gently.

I knew I must begin. "I've had a bit of a week … and I have some decisions to make."

His blue eyes looked at me. "Can I help?"

The wind breathed for me. "I don't know. I mean, yes … it's just that I had some minor surgery this week." I paused. "I've been told I have breast cancer."

The moment came and went. Peter looked stunned. His glance suspended the sky between us. He put his arm around my shoulder, and I slowly brought him up to date.

"It's nothing to worry about," I reassured Jenny at dinner. "Lots of women have breast cancer and it doesn't kill them." She remained uncharacteristically silent, so I continued, "The doctor wants to remove the breast just to make sure the cancer can't spread."

"What if it has already?" she asked.

"There are lots of other treatments available, lots of things that can be done," I said, hoping it was true. "Anyway, I don't know for sure that I'm going to have a mastectomy. It may not be necessary. There are other options, but I have to do some research first."

That night when I went to bed, Jenny climbed under the quilt and huddled up to me as she hadn't done since she was a very young child.

"Why do people have to die?" she asked.

I stroked her hair and answered her with a question. "Why do people exist? That's metaphysics," I said, and then added, "I'm not going to die. At least, not for a long time."

I held her close until she fell asleep. I found myself drifting back to blows I had received in my own childhood—the helplessness and agony of being separated from a parent—and I understood.

The next morning I went onto automatic pilot, planning the order in which certain things needed to happen. I called Katherine, who handled the news sensitively. She wanted to come home from university the next weekend, but I convinced her to wait until I had decided what to do.

I remembered that I had a midterm exam for one of my classes that night. At first, I felt there was no possible way I could study, and then I told myself, Just do it. By the time I got to class, I was convinced that I had enough knowledge of the material to do a reasonable job. And this was a time for a reasonable job to be applauded.

When the exam was over, I settled back in my seat for the lecture. We were studying film as the most important art of the twentieth century. That night we were to see two films by France's New Wave director Alain Resnais. The first one screened was *Night and Fog*, a graphically disturbing documentary of life in a concentration camp. The second, *Hiroshima, Mon Amour*, was directed by Resnais but written by avant-garde French novelist Marguerite Duras. I copied down the professor's words as I heard them: "The film should be considered in terms of inconsolable memory as well as humankind's self-destructiveness.... What blocks truth and the emerging of revelation is not forgetting but repression: *A living creature is a memory that acts.*"

Hiroshima, Mon Amour opened with the movement of two formless, anonymous shapes, like supple bodies, making love. Their skin glistened not with perspiration but with radioactive dust. The lovers were lost in their intimate embrace and seemingly savoured the ecstasies of the moment. Their love-making was accompanied by a dreamlike incantation of two voices. Although a man's voice responded, the film was a woman's story, written and told by a woman: "It's a matter of history … I didn't invent it…. So with Hiroshima, I had the illusion that one never forgets … just as in love."

I was mesmerized. It was a beautifully seductive combination of image, speech and sound. But then the film moved into harrowingly stark newsreel and documentary footage of the holocaust of Hiroshima. As I gaped at film footage of bald survivors with all their deformities, I felt as if more air than I could breathe had been forced into me.

The actress addressed "the impossibility of talking about humanity's crime against itself." She told her lover that indifference is the worst crime of all because "indifference makes history repeat itself." She explained how time and memory affect our sensibilities: if no one speaks out, we forget, and since it is our nature to be insensitive to what happens to others, what we know of as part of our past will be part of our future. "The art of seeing has to be learned," she said.

The savage loss of a past lover was a kind of personal Hiroshima for the actress. Just as she attempted to balance her own sorrow against the monumental tragedy, the dilemma of my own life reminded me of the universal significance of a much larger battle.

By the time I got home, Peter was already asleep. I moved near to him gently, so as not to wake him, but he put his arms around me. My breathing took on the rhythm of his.

I felt one of his hands travel down my back. I thought of Resnais's sensuous bodies slipping over and under each other, clasping and unclasping in swimming motions. I thought of the passion and dignity, the outburst of consciousness, the rise and fall of light and shade like alternate sensations. I thought how movies are the shadows of us all.

6

THE FIRST STARTLED MOMENT of waking became the most difficult for me. Not long ago, I had gone to sleep at night knowing I could wake up to greet the next day as it suited me. Now there was a certainty that this day, and all days to come, would be different from all the days of waking in the past.

At one of the most frightening moments of my life, I suddenly had to become a researcher and make cool decisions in a field I knew nothing about. It was not a likely time to be a smart consumer. I needed to focus on the treatment options so I could figure out which one or which combination was best for me: surgery to cut out the tumour, radiation to burn it or chemotherapy to poison it.

The whole thing seemed so unlikely. I didn't feel sick. I had always held on to my good health tenaciously, but now I was a woman caught on phrases like "riddled with it" or "died in battle." My fear was not so much of death—I was fond of living on the edge—but of the disease itself. As a paramedic, I knew that the progression of cancer was slow and dire, and that I must do everything I could to protect the people I loved from going through such a hellish experience.

I went ahead with all the medical tests. Blood tests to determine if the cancer had spread to my liver. An ultrasound and liver scan to help confirm those findings. A chest X-ray to determine whether or not the cancer had extended to my lungs.

I knew that all these tests would pick up only an advanced stage of cancer. Negative results didn't give anyone a clean bill of health; they simply indicated that there were no large tumours. There were no tests available to determine if microscopic cancer cells were elsewhere in the body.

When Dr. Harris first suggested I have a bone scan, I froze. "If the cancer has reached my bones, I'm out of here," I said.

"It's not because I believe the cancer is in your bones," he was quick to respond. "It will just give us a set of pictures to compare with, in case you start to develop new symptoms."

Reluctantly, I went off to the hospital's nuclear medicine department to have the scan. A technician injected a bone-seeking radioactive tracer into a vein in my arm. The objective was to have the tracer collect in any area of the bone where there was abnormal cell activity. It would take the phosphorous compound a while to travel through my bloodstream, so I had to wait a few hours for the actual "shoot."

To pass the time, I walked over to the hospital's ambulance station to talk with the crew members who were between calls. When I told them I was waiting for a friend who was undergoing some medical tests, they invited me to watch television with them. Isaac Stern was giving a concert in Jerusalem. But just as I sat down, sirens warned concertgoers of a Scud attack. The camera panned to the audience as every man, woman and child put on a gas mask. Then the camera roamed across the fleeing backs of the Israeli Philharmonic Orchestra musicians. Isaac Stern was left alone on the stage, playing a Mozart solo to an audience of humans with heads like ants.

I closed my eyes, registering the horror and the beauty simultaneously. It was all incomprehensible. One of the crew members switched to another channel. This station was reporting a massive air raid on Baghdad in which a two-thousand-pound laser-guided bomb had slammed into what the allies believed to be a command and control bunker. It had turned out to be packed with civilians, many of them children. There were close-up shots of the charred remains of countless unidentifiable people. The shelter had been reduced to rubble. A line from *Hiroshima, Mon Amour* flashed into my head: "It is our nature to be insensitive to what happens to others." I was startled to feel tears in my eyes. Without a word, I slipped out the door and took the most indirect route I could think of to the nuclear medicine department.

I had transported patients here by stretcher many times, but I had always left before the actual test took place. This time I was the patient. A technician instructed me to lie down on the cold metallic table of a machine that would take a picture of my entire skeleton. The scanner was pulled directly over my head. I was asked not to move. It made me feel claustrophobic, and I had to play a mind game to keep myself still. I breathed in—one, two, three—and breathed out. Slowly, the scanner started to travel towards my feet, so close that it was almost touching my skin. As it passed over me, it read the number of radioactive particles in the landscape of my body.

Once the test was completed, the technician told me that Dr. Harris had asked her to let me know if the results were negative. "Everything looks fine," she said.

I walked outside, breathing in the cold windy air like an addict high on a new drug. I unbuttoned my jacket and let it flap around me. "Everything looks fine." At least the cancer was not in an advanced stage in my bones. At least there was that.

I wanted to go home and kayak the high seas, but instead I set off for the Cancer Agency. Walking through the halls to the library, I nodded to some of the familiar nurses and doctors.

I headed towards a table in the corner and draped my jacket over the chair. The room was deadly quiet.

I booted up a cold computer, then did a search for all the articles that might provide me with the information I was after. After pulling some of the reports myself, I handed a list of those I couldn't find to the librarian. With an armful of papers and books, I sat down and got to work.

I learned that the incidence of breast cancer had increased 130 per cent in the past thirty years. One report said that if this increase continued at its current rate, in fifty years *every* North American woman over the age of thirty-five could expect to be diagnosed with breast cancer before the age of ninety-two. This year in North America, there would be almost 200,000 new diagnoses and more than 50,000 deaths. The report made a shocking comparison to put this number in perspective: 57,000 Americans had died in the nine years of the Vietnam War.

I did some quick arithmetic. On this continent alone, a woman was dying of breast cancer every ten minutes. Breast cancer was not only the leading killer of women aged thirty-five to fifty-four but also accounted for the largest "person-years of life lost" from all cancers—an average of twenty-two years per diagnosis. Even my job as a paramedic had not made me aware that breast cancer was an epidemic. How could this have happened? How could such a terrible disease not be known for the killer it was? If a flu were killing one person every ten minutes, it would make front-page headlines every day.

Was the disease still on the rampage simply because women had not spoken out, because we had been socialized not to complain? I knew from my work that women sometimes went to their graves without anyone but their doctors knowing they had breast cancer—because of the stigma attached to the disease, I suspected.

Although I came across numerous scientific reports, there was only the occasional paper written by a woman who had personally experienced a mastectomy. I found myself angry at the startling lack of information about a procedure that had been going on since the 1800s. I thought of all the stories that had been written about war and battlefields. Where were *our* stories?

One article argued that the cutting off of a woman's breast was a direct attack on the very symbols of femininity and eroticism celebrated by our society. Down the road was sure death. In the interim, the disease had the reputation of ruining one's love life, marriage or friendships, costing a promotion or even a job, and making it impossible to get health or medical insurance. It was small wonder that women tended to be secretive about it, I realized.

What shocked me, article after article, was how little anyone really knew about this disease. Medical researchers were mystified about why an increasing number of women were stricken every year. There were known causes for many other types of cancer, but researchers had no explanation for the cause of the initial genetic mutation that occurred with breast cancer, and no answers for the countless variables in the course the disease followed.

Why, for instance, was it impossible to predict the course and outcome of breast cancer once it was diagnosed? Why did women with the least favourable prognoses sometimes live many years longer than women diagnosed with what seemed to be small, contained tumours? And to what could the blame be attached?

I was amused by an article called "Breasts Beautiful." A plastic surgeon maintained that women were exhibiting a new breast fixation that exemplified a postfeminist expression of "self-assurance." He included pictures of Hollywood-style breasts: mountainous breasts, beehive breasts, eggplant breasts. Sculptures for love. All this voluptuousness sabotaged my research, and in my imagination I poured myself into a curve-clinging dress.

For the next two hours, I read without stopping about the treatment options available to me. My decision kept changing with each new piece of information I uncovered. Finally, frustrated, I leaned back in my chair. I closed my eyes and imagined three women joining me at my table: Dr. Surgeon, Dr. Radiation and Dr. Chemotherapy. Although I knew that in real life these doctors worked co-operatively with one another, helping patients to make decisions based on relative risks and benefits, in my head I set each of them up to play devil's advocate for her own form of treatment.

All three doctors agreed on one thing: surgery was the logical first attack on a malignant breast tumour. A modified radical mastectomy, the kind of surgery Dr. Harris had recommended, would remove the breast, the underarm lymph nodes and sometimes the lining over the chest wall. But there was growing evidence that a lumpectomy—the removal of the lump rather than the entire breast—might be preferable. On this issue, the doctors had different opinions.

Dr. Surgeon believed that *any* damage to my body was justified if it saved my life. But Dr. Radiation warned that the cut made into my tumour during the biopsy could have sent cancer cells into my bloodstream; there was the possibility that they might set up a secondary disease. And she believed that the anaesthetic I had been given—and was about to be given again—can suppress the immune system, allowing rapidly developing cells to gain a foothold in vulnerable scar tissue.

I squirmed in my chair. None of this was good news.

I let Dr. Surgeon argue. "My colleague will recommend that you be bombarded with her deadly rays, but she'll probably be reluctant to tell you that the treatment meant to cure also kills."

Dr. Radiation's answer was quick. "What my treatment can do is shrink or destroy a localized area of her cancerous cells *before* or *after* surgery."

"But radiation might also damage her other tissues and organs."

"A mastectomy is overkill."

"Radiation is simply not good for her."

"If she comes to me, there will be less disfigurement and she'll have the same statistical chance of survival."

"A mastectomy is more aggressive."

"A mastectomy *seems* more aggressive. A mastectomy will remove her breast tissue, but she may still have residual cancer cells in the area. I'll send her for surgery to have the rest of the tumour removed, then I'll radiate the whole breast area, killing any of those residual cancerous cells."

I knew I had to let Dr. Chemo have her turn. She said she could show me countless testimonials and case studies where women attributed their survival to radiation *and* chemotherapy. I decided to forget the other two doctors for the moment. "But," I said, "your treatments are horrific. No one would want to undertake them if they could possibly avoid it."

"I'm proud of what I do," Dr. Chemo argued. "My treatment can travel to the outreaches of your body where cancer cells may still be hiding. It's a search-and-destroy mission."

"What you're talking about is chemical warfare."

"It may seem unfortunate, but the more aggressive the treatment with chemotherapy, the better the chances for cure."

"The objective would be to poison my body to the limit of my tolerance. Admit it—your treatment simply *hopes* to reduce my risk of dying over the next five to ten years. It's band-aid stuff."

"Well, it's almost the year 2000, and at least I'm not still into knives and bloodletting."

"Dr. Surgeon's treatment won't weaken my immune system by killing off my white blood cells."

"Don't forget the effect of the anaesthetic—"

"If you were honest, you'd admit that you really don't know what I need—whether or not I should even have chemo, let alone which kind, for how long, which agents. All you can do is act on your hunches."

I slammed a book down on the table. The process of gathering information was like walking through a maze. I had to find the right way, but how? My work had made me all too aware of the human cost of surgical, radiation and chemotherapy errors or complications. Radiation and chemotherapy were relatively new treatments, and their long-term effects on the body were not known. A secondary cancer caused by radiation therapy did not appeal to me. And doctors and researchers seemed to agree that chemotherapy alone was not an option for destroying the cancer that already existed in my breast. Lumpectomy, along with radiation and possibly chemotherapy, appeared to be preferred to a mastectomy nowadays. A woman was believed to get the same results in terms of survival, and she got to keep her breast.

Because of the size of my tumour and its position, I had already had about a third of my breast removed. By the time all of the tumour—and a wide enough margin of tissue around it—was taken, it seemed to me that my breast wouldn't even look like a breast any more. A mastectomy was a mutilating choice, but I was dealing with a life-threatening disease. And in my particular case, mammograms had already proven useless for future detection.

I took a last glance at a page of statistics. One chart told me that 60 per cent of recurrences happened in the first three years after initial treatment; 20 per cent within the following two years; 20 per cent in later years. Another chart showed that 80 per cent of women with small tumours and no lymph node involvement made it past five years. I didn't know yet if I had node involvement, but I suspected I'd be disqualified from this group anyway because I had a large tumour.

There was so much to absorb and deal with. One foot in front of the other, I told myself. Deal with this challenge the way you have dealt with all challenges. Keep moving. Learn and grow from the experience. Take control. After all, I said to myself, a breast is not a vital organ.

It was dark by the time I left the library. I was overwhelmed with information and didn't feel I could possibly carry on a normal conversation, but I had promised Pat I'd stop by for a visit. Her home was right on my route to and from the city, and I often dropped in to see her. Today, as I pulled into the driveway, I saw her standing with an armful of firewood at the front door.

"Rosalind, my friend, where have you been hiding?" she shouted over a sudden gust of wind.

I followed her into the house. She threw the wood onto an already burning fire, then we gave each other a hug. I felt lost in her warmth, my body tired and heavy as if I hadn't slept for days.

"Is everything okay?" she asked, stepping back and assessing me with one eye closed.

"Sure," I replied inanely. "Why?"

"Well, you seem—" She paused, as if she couldn't find the word she wanted. "Everything's not okay, is it?"

I looked away. "Actually, I've found out I have breast cancer." I heard my voice trail off.

"Cancer," she repeated with slow deliberation. She shook her head and simply said, "Roz." She seemed to be beyond speech. Finally she said, "I'm so sorry. I'm in shock. I just don't know what to say."

"That's okay." I smiled at her. "I think I'm in shock too."

"How can I help?"

I leaned against the warm bricks of the fireplace. I was close to tears. "Just keep me from taking it all too seriously."

She hadn't taken her eyes off me. I tried to lighten things up a little. "As long as we can all keep a sense of humour, I'll survive this."

As if someone had pushed a button, Pat suddenly jumped into action, linking her arm through mine, steering me into the kitchen. "Come and sit down," she said. "This calls for a little drink."

"Not for me, thanks. I have a lot of decisions to make just now. I feel like I'm handling everything well except when I'm really tired or when I drink. Then I start to feel down."

"Small wonder," she said, pouring herself a tall vodka. "You know, Roz, when David and Tom were killed in the slide, we were a little overwhelmed by how much people wanted to help. And we didn't really know how to handle it. A *friend* told us that people have a need to help, and that it was our responsibility to let them do so."

She gave my old words a moment or two to sink in. Then she leaned across the table and placed her hand on mine. "You are going to have a lot of people who will want to help you. You must let them. After all the wonderful support you've given us, you know I will do anything."

She seemed to be waiting for a reply. I nodded a silent thank you.

"How long has all this been going on?"

"Two or three weeks, I guess. More than a month since I first felt the lump."

"What can I do?"

"I don't know. My mind is reeling."

"Who knows about this?"

"Only my family, and Deirdre."

"Then it's time," she said with a smile, "to go public." She poured herself another drink and continued, "Roz, I have a special favour to ask you—let me tell at least a few select people."

"I don't know, Pat. A few select people to you means dozens. For some reason, I don't want others to know."

She seemed not to buy it. "Roz, your friends will be very hurt if you don't let them know. And once they know, they will be devastated," she said, with a dramatic sweep of her hand. "So many people will need you to survive this—they will need *you* to help them through it."

"I don't know—I haven't decided what to do yet. I have a lot to learn before I can make decisions."

"But there's so much they can do about breast cancer nowadays."

I didn't know how to respond to that, so I said nothing.

She challenged me with her eyes. "Look at me."

I felt I was losing ground. "You are going to beat this thing," she said. "And you're going to let me go every step of the way with you. Okay?"

It always seemed easiest to give in to Pat. She was used to getting her way. I nodded acceptance of her terms. And as I did, I no longer felt as weary.

7

MY JOB HAD TAUGHT ME that keeping busy, and sticking to what is familiar, were effective techniques for dealing with terror. The next few days were lost to administrative duties: scheduling, reading memos, writing letters, ordering supplies. But underneath it all was an acute awareness of time on the fly.

I thought I had organized everything into manageable steps, but then one of Jenny's teachers called me at home to say that Jenny had been crying at school. "It's just not like her," the teacher said. "She normally has such a happy-go-lucky attitude towards everything—I thought you should know."

By the time I hung up, I had made my decision. I would go ahead with the mastectomy, but on my own terms. I phoned Dr. Harris's office and set up an appointment for later that day. I phoned an acquaintance who worked in the operating room at the hospital and asked her for the names of the three best anaesthetists she knew. No more luck of the draw. Next, I called my life insurance agent to make sure my policy was in order.

I sat at the table in front of our dining room window. The view framed by the large vertical window was like a photograph of a cheerless winter landscape. It had turned cold again. I craved sunshine and warmth. It occurred to me that the most important skill I had picked up in my early years was the ability to be somewhere else simply by staring out a window. I had endured then, and I would endure now. But what, I wondered, could I do for Jenny? Just in case our time together was to be short, I decided to create a special memory for her.

Dr. Harris's nurse, Nancy, took me right into the doctor's office. I noticed a framed family portrait on his desk. Like me, he had two daughters.

The office was very warm. Out a window I could see the bare limbs of a tree slowly turning white with snow. I heard the muted sounds of traffic from the street.

When the doctor came into his office, I laid out my decision. I gave him the names of the three anaesthetists and asked him to choose one. Then I told him I was taking my younger daughter out of school and leaving for Mexico for a week. My surgery would have to follow our trip.

He accepted my plan without argument. "You realize," he said, "that I'll also be doing a lymph node excision?"

"Yes."

"You understand why we do this?"

"To see if there is systemic involvement—if the cancer has spread beyond my breast."

"On the bright side," he said, "your tests have turned out clear, and nothing suspicious showed up in your bone scan."

I nodded.

"Now what we hope for is that it's non-metastatic, a cancer that hasn't moved from the place it started."

He pulled a book out of his desk drawer and started to show me pictures of breast reconstruction. The photographs made me feel ill. I looked away as he described the process. I could just make out a few of the words on the diplomas on the wall behind him.

I heard him say, "They are doing some wonderful work in reconstruction these days."

I could see how well they were doing. To me, it was a freak show. But I said nothing until he finished talking. Then I told him I would never want reconstruction. It was more surgery— very complicated surgery. It wouldn't be me. I understood that other women might feel differently. It just wasn't something I wanted for myself.

How quickly my life has changed, I thought, as I drove to my travel agent's office thinking of lymph nodes. The nodes that had once been my immunity, my certainty against infection, had become conspirators against me. My body had made a serious mistake.

I chose Mexico as our destination for several reasons. I had a pathological craving for sun, and Mexico was not too far away or expensive. The sultry climate induced a languor in everyone. But there was another important reason: Mexico's philosophy that life must be taken one day at a time and borne with fortitude and resilience. As soon as I had the plane tickets, I went on a shopping spree to buy clothing tailored with pockets over each breast. I smiled at myself as I bought sexy underwear. I called the doctor from a pay phone to give him my dates of travel. He said he would book the surgery for the day after our return.

"Just like that?" I asked. "No problem in booking that date?"

"Just like that," he said.

I hung up and headed for a restaurant where I had arranged to meet Deirdre and Pat. My eyes scanned the room but neither one of them had arrived yet, so I sat at a table and ordered myself a Kahlúa and milk.

Deirdre was the first to arrive. As she approached the table, her long black skirt stirred the air around her. She wore black with panache, but then she wore everything with panache.

I noticed that although her face was made up with care, she looked extraordinarily tired.

I put my hand up to greet hers. "How are you?" I asked.

She didn't answer, but flopped into a chair across the table from me and said in one breath, "God, what a day—how did it go for you?"

"You first," I answered, concerned.

She tossed a few loose strands of hair off her face and said, "Just family stuff. We're sorting through all my father's belongings. It's so depressing."

"Can I do anything?"

"No, but thanks. There are just so many memories." She ordered a glass of wine. "At least I've had this drink together to look forward to—it kept me going. So what's happening?"

"Well, on Sunday I'm taking Jenny to Mexico for a week and then I'm coming back to have a mastectomy."

She gazed at me like someone coming out of hypnosis. "Mexico? Why Mexico?"

"Sun and fun," I said cheerfully. "Just in case I have only ten minutes left to live, I want Jenny to have this experience with me."

Deirdre smiled feebly. "Roz, we *all* have only ten minutes left to live."

My entire body went on the alert, and I searched her face. At first I thought she had spoken lightly, but I could see from her expression that she was very serious. Something heavy slid from my logical mind down into my heart and anchored there.

We were silent for a moment, sipping our drinks. "Hey, wait a minute—*when* are you leaving?" she said suddenly.

"Who's going where?" Pat leaned over to embrace me and then Deirdre.

"I am," I said with renewed cheer.

"Okay, start at the beginning and don't miss a detail. It sounds like you've made some decisions."

I waited while she ordered her drink, and then I informed her of my plans.

Pat placed her hand lightly on my wrist. "Wonderful," she said. "What a perfect way to do it."

"I think so," I said.

I looked at Deirdre, but her thoughts appeared to be elsewhere. I nudged her gently with my foot. "What's the problem?" I asked.

"That trip we've been planning—I'll be in Hawaii when you're having surgery," she groaned. "Everything is booked. The whole family is going. I had no idea your surgery could happen so quickly."

"Not to worry." I smiled, pushing aside a feeling of disappointment. I knew it would be good for her to get away.

"You know how long we've been planning this trip—"

"Deirdre, honest, it's okay. I'll miss you, but I'll survive."

Pat looked troubled all of a sudden. "What if you get one of those intestinal things while you're in Mexico? Do you think maybe you should do the trip after the surgery?"

"No, I'll be careful."

Deirdre let out a loud sigh. "When did you say you leave?"

"Sunday," I said.

"If we hadn't already paid for the tickets—"

"I'll tell you what—if I need chemotherapy, you can help me find a wig when you get back."

We all laughed at the idea. I put my hands behind my head as if displaying a new hair-do. "Maybe I'll be a redhead for a change. Or perhaps dark and mysterious?"

"A Madonna look," Pat suggested, then added wickedly, "Whoops, we might have a little trouble with the *other* part of your body."

We laughed, finished off our drinks and walked out into the icy edge of a winter wind.

On my way home, I thought of Deirdre's comment about everyone having only ten minutes left to live. It was a peculiar thing to say to someone who had recently been told her cells had gone berserk. But I reminded myself that at the moment she was stretched to her emotional limit. She had probably just been trying to normalize the situation.

I stopped at the ambulance station. Jeff, who had often been acting chief when I was away, was huddled against the building, smoking a cigarette.

I smiled as I approached. "I thought you quit," I said.

He grinned back. "I did, but you know how it is."

I leaned against the wall beside him, rubbing my cold hands together. "Jeff, you've done such a good job of running the station when I've been away before—would you mind doing it for another month or so?"

"Sure," he said, grinding the cigarette out with his foot. "You off to someplace?"

"Mexico," I said.

"For a month?"

"Actually, for a week." I paused. "I've recently found out I have breast cancer. The day after I get back from Mexico, I will be going into the hospital for a mastectomy."

He leaned forward so abruptly that he almost fell over. "You're not kidding, are you?"

"No, I'm not. And if you don't mind, I'd prefer if it wasn't advertised all over the place."

"Of course. I understand."

"Don't you dare write me off," I said, pointing my finger at him.

"Not a chance. This place falls apart without you."

"Thanks," I said.

"Can I do anything?"

I nodded and waved for him to follow me. "Let's go inside and I'll show you what needs to be done."

As soon as I had finished going through the paperwork with Jeff, the ambulance went out on a call. I tidied up my desk and picked up a few leaves that had fallen from a ficus tree by the window.

I'd been very upbeat with Jeff. All the crew members were used to seeing me that way. It was an image I worked at; I was proud of being perceived as someone able to bear up no matter what the challenge. After all, I had everything: an interesting job, success as a published poet, an eventful life with great friends. I had a home that was my special spot on earth. And I had a husband and two daughters whom I loved not only as a woman loves her family but because of the kind of people they were.

It could be worse, I convinced myself. Much worse. My breasts had brought me great pleasure before and after marriage. I'd had the joy of nursing both my children, who were grown up enough to cope on their own if they had to. I couldn't imagine the terror a woman in my situation must go through if her children were very young.

From *have* to *have not*. No more breasts to the wind. I packed for Mexico and the blessed relief of sun.

We arrived in Puerto Vallarta. As we made our way through customs, an airport official asked, "What kind of trip? Business or pleasure?"

"Pleasure," I answered. But it's really unfinished business, I thought.

"Okey-dokey," he said, looking at our passports and waving us forward.

For the first few days, Jenny and I did little more than take our slowly bronzing bodies to the beach. We played endlessly in the waves. They seemed to come in varying sets—a series of a half-dozen or so small waves followed by the same number of large ones. What was deceiving was the apparent quiet between the sets of waves. That was when a huge, unexpected one might flatten you. Needing to protect the dressings covering my incision, I was a little meek compared with Jenny, who on some occasions came up out of the water without the top of her two-piece bathing suit.

Some good-looking Mexican youths watched with amusement. They warned us never to turn our backs to the sea. "That will be when the big one hits—we call them sleepers."

It was a wonderfully lazy and dreamlike week. We never once discussed my diagnosis. Although I was constantly reminded of what lay ahead by my physical discomfort and the surgical dressings, my fear was pushed aside by laughter and sunshine, horseback riding, parasailing and renting jeeps for photography expeditions.

The hot land pulsed—systole, diastole—that tomorrow was another day.

Peter was waiting at the airport. We held on to each other for a long time. "You two look like you've had a ball," he said, delighted.

As he drove us home, Jenny and I filled him in on our week.

"Katherine will be writing an exam tomorrow," he said, as

he turned off the highway and headed up the hill. "She's coming home the day after that."

"She shouldn't be coming home at exam time."

"She says she wants to. I think her mind is made up."

"What about exams?" I pushed him, wanting more information.

"She said to tell you it's her decision." He glanced sideways at me. "She said she needs to be with you right now."

I worried about Katherine missing classes, but I was secretly happy to hear she would be home. I looked at my watch. It was past midnight, already Monday. "I guess it's a little late to be calling her in residence, isn't it?"

"I think so. You'll see her soon," he said. "Here we are, home."

Coming out of my shower that night, I stood naked in front of the mirror and tried to imagine what I might look like after tomorrow. I couldn't.

I tried on the elegant white bathrobe Pat had bought for me to wear in the hospital. It set my tan off nicely. "Hmmm," I said quietly to the woman in the mirror. "If tomorrow is an event, you might as well look good when it happens."

It was two o'clock by the time I made it to bed. Except for my small dressings, I was naked. I lay down on our mattress. We still hadn't got around to buying a bed, and in the meantime we'd decided we didn't want more than a mattress on the floor. Looking out the window, I could see enormous dark mountains above me, and beyond that a clear, starlit night sky.

Peter was still awake. We held each other close. I moved my face away from his, and he kissed me. I could feel the muscles of his shoulders through his pyjama top. I started to undo the buttons. I felt his chest next to my breasts. I felt so alive as we rose and fell, rose and fell into the darkness.

In the morning Jenny watched me pack. "Do you want to take a picture of us with you?" she asked.

I thought of Maggie. "No, I want you guys there in the flesh."

I stopped and looked at my daughter. She was brown-skinned and gleaming as if she had been polished by the sun. "Are you okay?"

With a grim smile, she nodded.

"Good, because I'm okay too. You're coming to visit me after school?"

"After work," she smiled. "I promised someone at the coffeehouse that I'd cover for her today. Just for a couple of hours. Then I'll bring in our pictures from Mexico."

As we were about to go out the door, the phone rang, sharp and cheerful. I ran back upstairs.

Although it was a bad connection, I instantly recognized Deirdre's voice.

"I'm so glad I got hold of you," she said.

"Hey, how is Hawaii?" I asked.

"Actually, I'm standing in a telephone booth in the rain."

"God, I hope it's warm rain."

"Listen, I was scared I'd miss you. I just wanted you to know I'm thinking about you. I know everything will go well but ... I wish I were there."

"Thanks, Deirdre. We're just heading to the hospital."

"Mexico work out for you?"

"It was fabulous. One of the best weeks of my life."

"Good. Hang in there. Promise me that."

"You can count on it. But you have to promise me *you'll* have a good time."

"I will," she said. "Good luck."

"Thanks, Deirdre," I said across the miles. "Thanks for calling."

I hung up and looked out at the water, where upside-down mountains reached for the blue sky beneath them. I missed Deirdre already.

Freyja watched attentively, cocking her head from one side to the other.

"No, my friend, you're not coming along," I told her. I bent over to wrap my arms around her neck. "Keep my side of the bed warm," I whispered, giving her one more pat on the head.

We dropped Jenny off at school on our way to the hospital. It was less then twenty hours since she and I had been on the beach in Puerto Vallarta, and it was not going to be an easy day for her. But I felt tanned, fit and healthy. I was as ready as I could ever be.

Waiting to be admitted, I let my gaze drift over all the people walking in and out of the automatic doors. Once again, as a patient, I became part of the impersonal and clinical hospital environment. I was dependent on strangers. I leafed through a magazine article; new research suggested that cancer was the byproduct of stress.

"Can you believe it?" I exclaimed to Peter. "I've always thought I thrived on stress." The article said that mastectomies were rarely done nowadays, and that a postoperative depression could be expected by all women who had one. Not me, I thought: I'm doing just fine.

As soon as the paperwork was completed, we took the elevator to a ward on the fourth floor. There were three women in the room. The woman in the bed directly across from mine was asleep. At a glance, I could tell she was cadaverously thin. I smiled and nodded at the other two, and they smiled back. The woman in the far corner was talking to someone, probably her husband. She had a very loud voice.

A nurse breezed into the room. "How are you, Mrs. MacPhee?"

"Fine, thank you," I said, matching her enthusiasm.

She asked me to change and showed me where I could put my things.

"Maybe I should go now?" Peter suggested. I nodded, sensing that he felt he might be in the way. "I'll come back later," he said.

"No need," I said. "Jenny wants the car so she can come for a visit. If you're as tired as I am, you should be going home after work for a good night's sleep."

We wrapped our arms around each other and just stood there for a moment. I could feel his heart beating fast.

I pulled the curtains around my bed and changed. I put away the few things I'd brought with me: Jenny's Walkman, tapes of Bach, Corelli, Scarlatti and Satie, notes to study in preparation for my final exam. For relaxation, I had Joan Didion's *Play It as It Lays* and Wilkie Collins's *The Woman in White*. The significance of the titles wasn't lost on me.

I felt silly in a hospital gown. I wasn't sick—I'd never felt better. I wrapped myself in the luxurious white robe that Pat had given me, feeling like a guest who had arrived too early. I sat down in the chair beside the bed and propped my study notes on my lap. I stared at the words. I read the same lines over and over again. Nothing was sinking in.

A delivery man came into the room bearing flowers. The card read, "With love from Brenda and family." More flowers arrived—I suspected that Pat had been busy while I was away. She sent a huge, heroic-looking plant with a long, impossible-to-say name.

Nurses came and went from the room, taking vitals, writing information on my chart. But for the most part I was ignored, and I wondered why they had wanted me there that early. I sat in the chair for so long that I started to look to the window for signs of oncoming darkness. The words to a song buzzed in my head, "Don't let the sun go down on me …"

It was late afternoon when a nurse came in and introduced herself as Marie. "Had your bath yet?" she asked.

"I had a shower late last night and another one early this morning." I smiled at her.

"You'll need another one, I'm afraid. Then I'll need to shave under your arm."

I hadn't thought of that. I wondered how many other things I hadn't thought of. But I did as I was asked.

When Marie came back, she asked me to lie on the bed while she shaved me. She glanced at my notes on the table. "Are you studying for something?"

"Yes, I'm trying to finish off my degree—it's taken me twenty years, so I can't quit now."

"But can you concentrate? The night before surgery?"

"Actually, I've been reading the same line over and over all day," I confessed.

"Oh," she said, nodding. "Well, I saw you reading away earlier and I was amazed. Usually women come in here and stare at a wall or the ceiling." She patted me on the shoulder. "After dinner, I'll come back and give you a nice back rub. If you like, we'll talk."

I lay on top of the bed and closed my eyes, trying to find my centre, to ground myself. The smell of dinner floated in the room. When my tray arrived, I peeked under the plastic cover to see if I could identify the food.

A woman dressed in hospital greens appeared beside my bed. She introduced herself as my anaesthetist. "I'm sorry to interrupt your dinner, but I'd like to ask you a few quick questions."

"Certainly," I said, pushing my tray away.

"I read in your chart that you're a paramedic," she started conversationally.

"Yes," I said. My profession as a paramedic bred a respect, a kind of bond, with other medical people. I'd seen it happen many times before. People connected with the health system tended to get better care in a hospital. It shouldn't be that way, but there it was.

"This must be quite an experience for you. Being a patient, I mean. Do you have any questions regarding your surgery?"

"You know how to start an IV? The last anaesthetist blew more starts than we're allowed when we're working at the side of the road in the dark of night in the middle of a blizzard."

She lifted my left arm, turned it over and ran her fingers gently over my veins. "Has anyone had trouble starting a line on you before?"

"Never—one pop and you're in."

"Well, your last surgery was scheduled to happen early in the day but ended up late in the afternoon. Sometimes people get dehydrated and tense when they have to wait so long. Their veins go flat."

She was a professional, and she was trying to excuse one of her colleagues. I let her get away with it.

"I also tend to throw up after surgery," I said.

"That's not necessary. I can give you something so that doesn't happen."

She looked around the room. "Would you like something to help you sleep tonight? It's not a bad idea, particularly when you're in a ward."

I didn't answer at first. But then I decided that only a fool would say no to an offer like that in a place like this.

Jenny arrived with our photographs of Mexico and a photograph album. We spent several hours immersed in reliving our trip as we placed the pictures on the pages. We talked about the sound of the cicadas at night. We talked about all the young Don Juans. We talked about deserted beaches, deep white sand, the crashing sea. We talked about everything except the next morning's surgery. She stayed very late. It was only when she left that the hours grew long enough for my thoughts to wander.

I reflected on what I had valued most in my life. Two things came to my mind: the people I loved, and the trips I had taken into the wilderness. I found it interesting that all else seemed unimportant: the work that was so meaningful to me, the writing that so often obsessed me and even the home where I had lived for so many years.

Despite the sedative they'd given me, I found it impossible to fall asleep. Countless times I flipped the pillow under my head. I was aware of the smallest sounds: nurses murmuring in the hall, someone turning over in bed, a distant siren. Marie came in and pulled up a chair beside my bed. I thought of all the hands I had held in my job and readily accepted the one she offered.

Early the next morning, I was prepared for surgery. I slipped into the surgical gown, leg-warmers and hair net. I was given something in a small paper cup to neutralize my stomach acid. I felt quite relaxed, and wondered if they'd put a bit of Valium in the small cocktail I'd swallowed.

I had to wait for some time before being moved to the operating room. I thought of an expression of comfort Peter and I had picked up from a television program: "Never mind, love, we'll have a nice cup of tea." Saying this was an important ritual for us. It was our way of recognizing the fact that we had managed in one way or another to survive together. I knew that if he were here right now, that's what he'd be saying.

Finally, an orderly wheeled me down halls covered in green tile. He pushed my stretcher through swinging doors to a waiting population of masked people. Nurses strapped me onto a high, narrow bed in a windowless room. The room was cold. The coldness seemed to make it more difficult to prepare myself mentally for the physical assault that was to come.

I thought of how—not so long ago—operating rooms must have had windows. A patient might have heard a bird in a nearby tree or felt the warmth of the sun through a window. In this place, the sun was a large overhead fixture. Its glare was almost blinding. An automated blood pressure cuff was attached to my right arm. The needle for an intravenous was slipped into my other arm almost before I knew it was happening.

Dr. Harris commented, "That went in easily."

"Maybe it's because women are better with needles," I suggested.

"No, it's because you've now got the best hands in the business doing it."

I watched slow, repetitive drips of cold fluid head towards my vein. A small metal clip was attached to the end of one of my fingers. Someone explained that it was used to measure the amount of oxygen in my blood.

My green gown was unfastened at the neck, exposing my upper body to the coldness. I confirmed that the lump was in my right breast, and a nurse made a note on my chart. A sheet was folded neatly across my abdomen. Someone started to paint my right breast in a wide, circling pattern with an anti-septic the colour of fuchsias. My chest and upper arm were painted too. Small square towels were placed around the painted breast, then clipped together. I was draped with a large sheet—all of me except my right breast, which presented itself through an octagonal hole in the drape.

There was a large clock on the wall. It showed the time as 12:00. Noon. I set my mental clock to zero. I glanced at my breast and then looked back at the clock. It still showed 12:00. It seemed frozen in that position, like a clock rescued from some disaster recording the exact hour of the catastrophe.

I thought of mountains I had climbed, and alpine meadows. I closed my eyes and saw white sands drop sharply to a roaring sea. The electronic echo of the rhythm of my heart faded.

8

I DRIFTED IN AND OUT of consciousness. Someone gave me a shot of morphine whenever I woke up. My doctor was there but wasn't there. I wanted only to lie on my back. My right arm was propped up on something. In sleep, I was lost in a primal sea of images that I would later write down: *A matrix of blue glass ... the sky reflected fathoms deep ... a rush of sunlight deeper than water ... the deep pull of the migration ... the ocean's blue ambiguity ... as minnows move in hypodermic schools.*

I became aware that Peter was sitting beside my bed. Whenever I woke up, he was there. Quiet. Watchful. Sometimes holding my hand. His hand felt warm. A sensuous warmth moved up my arm and spread through me: *In the first light of morning, you fall on me like waves upon a shore ... as the sea glides in, light strokes my thighs, draws them apart ... we swim naked, move like water, the slow rise of longing in the wave of sunlight I wake to.*

Whenever I came out of the world of sleep, everyone told me that I radiated a sense of well-being. Pat visited. She said something to me about the sun, sealing the illogic of what she'd said with a kiss on my cheek.

They had intubated me during surgery—put a tube down my throat to my lungs. My throat wasn't all that sore, but when I spoke, I didn't recognize my voice.

A day or two passed. Peter still sat in a chair beside me. I wondered if he had gone home and come back again. I was aware of a great deal of pain, but I was also on a high from the morphine. I knew that the drug had an amnesic effect. It was a great blocker of reality: *Light approaches so perceptibly. It might be a tide line, or pain too close. There is this slow arousal. The surgical sun amazingly bright throws its light onto my bed. It makes me tremble: wet. I am startled by its urgent rhythms. I feel its violence shudder in my hands. It pulls back my covers and takes me from behind, moaning that it cannot stop ... will not stop ... filling my body warm like water while I move with the slow practised strokes of a swimmer.*

At first, a nurse assisted me whenever I asked to go to the bathroom; although I felt weak, I had no great difficulty getting there. I was kept on an intravenous, and there were suction devices with tubes inserted beneath the dressings. Fluids that looked like watermelon juice were draining from the incision.

I was soon up and about on my own. I'd remove the IV bag from its pole and thread it through the sleeve of my robe, rehanging it with experienced hands. Although I felt I was carrying my right shoulder lower than my left, walking around was fine as long as I didn't try to go too far. It was the process of getting up from a lying position that was a challenge. I had to roll onto my left side to get out of bed. I began to wonder if I would ever lie on my right side again.

Cards and flowers surrounded me. There were serious cards and funny ones. There was a card with a picture of a mountain on it signed by everyone at Search and Rescue. There was another with a picture of a classy lady on the front. Inside I read, "Mexico I can understand, even Paris would be nice, Aruba is great any time ... but the hospital? I'd get a new travel agent if I were you. Love, Sylvia." Pat had also dropped off a card: "My reasons for wanting you to get well are really quite selfish—when you hurt, I hurt. Please get well soon." I read my cards, drifted asleep and then read them again when I awoke.

Outside my window, the Japanese cherry trees were blossoming. Yet it had turned cold, and snow had started to fall. The branches of the cherry trees were bent almost to breaking. For what seemed to be an eternity, I watched snow catch in the corners of the windows.

I woke to the sound of a stranger's quiet voice. "He maketh me to lie down in green pastures: he leadeth me beside the still waters .... Yea, though I walk through the valley of the shadow of death ..."

A priest held a closed Bible in his hand as he recited The Lord Is My Shepherd to the patient in the bed across the room. I had nicknamed her Mississippi; her name was something like Mrs. Sieppe, and I'd heard several different pronunciations of it.

Cancer seemed to be spreading into Mississippi's brain. She was often confused. Although she got up from time to time, she shuffled awkwardly down the halls as if acting under instructions. She moved so slowly that she made a sweeping sound.

I heard her ask the priest to read more psalms. A Bible reader I was not, but I enjoyed the language and imagery. I drifted in and out of sleep to the rise and fall of its music.

Word of my surgery had obviously reached friends—they arrived in droves. Pat came bustling in every day. And so did Donna, who had undergone a lumpectomy several years before. She brought me a copy of Bernie Siegel's book *Love, Medicine and Miracles*, which she said had been helpful to her.

Sylvia brought a stuffed animal—a frog. "It's a cancer-cell eater," she explained. During a very difficult time she'd had with cancer years earlier, someone had given her a cell-eating frog. She explained that she couldn't bear to give hers away and so had gone on a search for a look-alike.

She dangled the long-legged creature in the air. "It's important that he's very ugly," she said. "Keep him close and he'll devour any leftover cancer cells."

The visits of family and friends became my centre of gravity. The ward looked like a florist's shop; there was every sort of flower in the brightest of colours. I was touched by all the generous and thoughtful acts. They were the things I thought of as I drifted in and out of sleep.

The sound of a curtain being drawn woke me. Marie was on duty, offering a back rub.

I nodded towards Mississippi. "How is she doing?"

"She's dying," Marie said quietly.

I was lying on my left side, using my good arm as a pillow. I looked up at Marie. "Why isn't she in palliative care?"

"She used to be a nurse. To her, that ward is *the end*. She made her doctor promise never to put her there. It won't be long until she doesn't know where she is—I guess she'll be moved then."

We were interrupted by Dr. Harris, who came in to check my dressings. After a quick look, he pulled a chair up beside my bed, sitting on it the wrong way around with his arms resting on the metal back. His eyes were clear, grey and kind.

He told me that some of the lab work was back and that the type of carcinoma I had was a "common garden variety." Because the tumour had been large and some of the nodes were swollen, he had removed "everything that wasn't nailed down."

His eyes roamed back and forth to the flowers. "More waiting, I'm afraid, until the lab can tell us about the nodes." He smiled in a supportive way.

"How's the pain?" he asked, placing the chair back in the corner.

"Okay for the first two hours after morphine. Then I can't wait for the next shot."

"I'll look at your chart and see if we can up the dose. Don't try to use that arm yet," he warned. "Be patient, or you'll end up with some problems that will be a real nuisance to you later. Eventually we'll send you to physiotherapy, but for now just do whatever seems comfortable."

He took a last look at the dressings. I looked too. "You sure you did the surgery?" I asked. "With all the dressings I still feel symmetrical."

"You've had enough leakage to prove we did the job. We'll take these old dressings off tomorrow and give you some fresh ones." He waved and disappeared out the door.

Tomorrow, I said to myself. I hadn't thought it would be so soon.

The patient in the opposite corner of the ward was a huge, heavy-set woman, about fifty years old. I'd heard her called Jessie. She flaunted a ring with diamonds big enough to make me think of ice cubes. They flashed across the room as she filed and refiled her nails.

The woman in the bed beside me told me her name was Shannon. She was twenty-six years old, and she'd had a mastectomy five days before mine. She had just been told that she needed chemotherapy followed by six weeks of radiation. She was a schoolteacher with three children under the age of eight.

"I don't have time for breast cancer," she said, smiling just a little. "I'm really pissed off about it. I canvass for cancer research and thought I'd be spared."

The thought of going through all of this with the responsibility of young children at home made me shiver. But I laughed and said, "Life doesn't work that way."

"So it appears." She sighed. "But let me tell you something really scary. My mother had breast cancer and died from it when I was very young. My father tells me that the treatments I've been offered are exactly the same treatments she was offered, and that was twenty years ago. Haven't we learned anything in twenty years?"

Sometimes I wondered if choosing the interaction and company of others in a ward had been a mistake. It was most challenging at night. Mississippi often talked in her sleep, and Jessie would shout at her for doing it.

One night as I lay awake I heard Mississippi moving her dentures back and forth, and I knew she was up to something. Her feet shuffled across the floor. The next thing I knew she was looking down at me in the semidarkness. I saw her eyes swimming behind the thick lenses of her glasses.

"Willy," she said, startling me. "It's me. Move over, Willy."

"Mrs. Sieppe, I'm not Willy," I explained softly, pushing the call button for a nurse.

The beam of a flashlight swept the room, and a nurse gentled Mississippi by the elbow. "Mrs. Sieppe, this isn't your bed, love. Come along now."

I heard Shannon roll over and sigh, "Oh, God."

The nurse put the railings up on Mississippi's bed and tried to persuade her to take a sleeping pill. She came back to me and asked, "Anything I can get for you, Mrs. MacPhee?"

I had begun to sweat. "I could use another shot."

She nodded. "Is it morphine you need, or do you think a sleeping pill might do the trick?"

I requested morphine, knowing I must be close to the time of my next needle. The drug would also make me drowsy, I thought. Even so, I lay wide awake. I knew I wasn't the only one. Out of left field, Shannon said, "I'm glad my mother is dead."

I turned my head to look at her.

"A mom would be the hardest to tell."

I lay waiting for light, people and sound.

Early in the morning, an orderly came for Jessie. I wished her luck as she was wheeled out on a gurney.

Shannon slowly sorted through her things. Her doctor had told her she could go home. She saw me watching her fold her nightie into a small suitcase. "I don't feel so much like a patient when I wear my own nightgown," she explained.

Mississippi started to snore loudly enough that Shannon had to stand beside my bed so we could hear each other. She grinned at the older woman. "She's something else, isn't she?" Without waiting for a reply, she continued, "Apparently most people like to die at home. Did you know that? Would you want to die in a hospital or at home?"

Not liking the choice she'd given me, I said, "Somewhere else, I think."

She broke off a few spent flowers from one of my plants, and smiled. "The room smells like a garden. Where did all this stuff come from?"

"Friends and family," I replied. "A lot came from people in Lions Bay—that's where I live."

"But why so much?"

"Because they're neighbours."

She mulled this over briefly. "So who are you? Someone famous?"

Pat appeared in the doorway, hardly visible behind a huge arrangement of new flowers. She put the vase down with a great clunk, giving me a wink and telling Shannon, "No, not famous—just someone greatly loved."

Shannon laughed. "You must be one of those Lions Bay people."

"Actually, no," Pat said, looking as determined as I'd ever seen her. "I used to live in Lions Bay. I'd love to live there again. Unfortunately, they won't let me return because I left the place in such a mess."

I laughed, full of admiration for Pat's survival strategies.

Shannon's husband arrived and helped her into her jacket. Coming over to say good-bye, she added, "I hope everything works out for you."

I nodded. "You too, Shannon."

"Well, my mother didn't last a year after her breast cancer was diagnosed," she said, answering a question I didn't think I'd asked. "She had 'c.a.' in the liver—case closed. Then it hit her brain." Shannon glanced towards Mississippi. "My mother got just like that—*non compos mentis*."

"I'll tell you something else," she said, looking at Pat and me. "Humankind is toxic. These tumours are just evening the score. And I'm not leaving this world until I've blamed someone for nuclear testing, DDT, food additives ... all of it. That much I promise."

She glanced uneasily around the room. "Listen, don't go crazy in here. A person could, you know."

In a brief, conspiratorial way, we gave each other a hug.

"See you in politics," I said.

She posed dramatically in the doorway and made a plucky thumbs-up gesture.

Pat left shortly afterwards. I closed my eyes. When I opened them again I heard the voice of the priest say, "What thou seest, write in a book ..." He was thumbing through Revelations, sometimes reading and sometimes talking quietly to Mississippi. Jessie had returned from surgery. She was staring up at the little television set but glared from time to time at the priest, who occasionally smiled at her.

I pretended I had fallen back to sleep. Before the priest left, I heard him walk over to Jessie and ask, "And how are you?"

"Still on the right side of the grass, Reverend," she answered.

"Well, that's better than the alternative now, isn't it?" he answered good-humouredly. He wished her good day on his way out.

It wasn't long before I heard Jessie's voice. "Mrs. MacPhee, are you awake?"

"Yes."

"Did you hear him? He was trying to start a conversation! I don't want any reverend talking to me about the fate of the damned."

I looked at Mississippi. Her face had clouded over. She eyed us both but said to Jessie, "May God forgive you."

Jessie sat up straighter, pushing her small television set aside. "Hey, listen here. I think it's about time that God asks *us* to forgive *him*."

I raised my voice and asked Jessie, "How did your surgery go?"

She leaned back in defeat. "They want me stay here and have it lopped off. I can't believe it. I knew this would happen. Why couldn't they have just taken it off while I was out cold?"

"Well, that might be what you'd like, but lots of women want to know what they're dealing with before they lose a breast. I'm sure your doctor has told you there are other options."

"Sure, but once you have cancer, you just want the thing off so everything can get back to the way it was. Didn't you?"

"I suppose, in a way. But I certainly considered the other possibilities."

"The doctor says I have a kind of cancer that is called cluster, or star, or something like that. He says it's all through the breast."

I had to struggle to find something reassuring to say. "I've read that the *kind* of breast cancer you have doesn't have a lot to do with your chance of survival."

Jessie looked at me skeptically. "Yeah?" She turned away, staring silently at the television.

A flower arrangement in an ambulance urinal was suddenly thrust in front of me. Brian and Darcy, in uniform, stood behind it.

"In case you're missing work," they informed me. They brought me up to date on what was happening at the station and described some of the more interesting calls they'd recently attended. Brian talked about a naked man who had jumped two floors from his apartment building in a suicide attempt. "The poor guy must have figured it was run, jump, dead—but he was hardly injured."

Darcy interrupted. "It must have been one of those days when he couldn't do anything right."

Darcy, for his part, had gone to a call where a woman had been assaulted by another woman. He'd opened an apartment door, and there on a green shag rug lay a woman with a rabbit sitting on her stomach. There were a dozen or so rabbits in the apartment, soundlessly jumping in all directions.

I smiled. I could picture it all. Life, it seemed, went on.

I walked them to the elevators, pushing the spindly IV pole along beside me. As soon as they were gone, I went back to my room and stood at the window. The snow had disappeared; the weather was sunny. This time last year, I was on the other side of the country taking a course in disaster management. This was a different kind of disaster. A personal one.

I saw Brian and Darcy leave the hospital. My window overlooked the Emergency entrance, and I watched as ambulances glided in and out of the bay. It was the world I had come from so recently, yet it seemed incredibly remote. I stayed there until Darcy and Brian's ambulance pulled away.

Tomorrow, the dressings would be removed. I looked at my two hands, my two legs, and told myself I was ready.

9

A NURSE APPEARED IN THE DOORWAY, bringing in another patient to fill Shannon's bed. The woman was about my age and very anxious. I walked the halls while she changed and settled into hospital routine. When I came back she was sitting on her bed looking puzzled.

I introduced myself. "Hi, I'm Rosalind." She shook my hand

and smiled such a warm smile that it concealed any fear hiding behind it.

"Liz Berry," she said.

"Your first time in hospital?"

"Yes." She smiled. "I suppose I've made that obvious. But I feel like this is judgement day. I'm a lawyer, and I have a reputation for being formidable in a showdown. At the moment I'm trying to stave off panic."

"Habeas corpus." I smiled at her.

She laughed. "Whatever happened to plea bargaining? Gone is the feeling that 'they can't do nuthin' to ya.'"

"Are you in for surgery?"

She nodded.

"Well, I've had surgery and I'm on the mend. So if I can do anything, just let me know."

"Do you mind if I ask what kind of surgery you had?"

"A mastectomy," I said, aware that it was the first time since my surgery that I had spoken the word.

"Oh, my God," she said. "You look … you look so healthy and well."

"But I am," I assured her, smiling.

"That's why I'm here, too," she said quietly. "And I admit to feeling quite overwhelmed."

"I was too. But I'm sure it will go as well for you as it has for me." I did a few quick little steps with my feet. "Look, I can even dance."

We were both laughing when her husband walked into the room. I recognized him immediately as a police officer I often interacted with on the job. We said hello to each other, then I excused myself, closing the curtain between our beds to give them some privacy.

From the small amount I'd exerted myself, my body felt as

though it had plunged through a windshield. I was drenched with perspiration. When the nurse eventually arrived with a needle, she squinted at me. "My goodness, are you in that much pain?"

"There's room for improvement." I attempted a smile.

The morphine began to slowly flood through my body. I started to relax, asleep before she'd even left the ward. I didn't wake up until it was time for the next shot. The dinner trays arrived, and I was surprised at how hungry I felt. A nurse brought me a list of visitors who had come in while I was sleeping. "You know," she said, "we could put up a No Visitors sign for you."

"No, no," I said quickly. "I love the visits. I think maybe I need to cut a mile or two off my hall marathons. It's just that I'm scared of getting out of shape."

"Give yourself some time," she suggested. "You're doing wonderfully well. Right now you need to rest."

My only visitors that evening were my family. Jenny commented that I looked tired, and I watched Peter and Katherine nod in agreement.

"A little," I admitted. "I've been doing too much."

They left soon after, and I was asleep in no time. The next thing I was aware of was a moaning sound. I knew it was Mississippi. I heard her say to the darkness, "Who is that moaning? Could they please stop?"

Jessie bellowed at her, "It's you, you idiot. You've woken yourself up with your own moaning."

I wrapped my arms around myself, as though some awful cold had come into the room. Unable to sleep, I put on the head-phones for Jenny's Walkman. I listened to Glenn Gould play the Goldberg Variations. I heard the notes deeply, then distantly, as I was carried away by Bach.

The sun on its rounds—the room suddenly flooded with light. The bustle of hospital routine had started again. Temperatures and vitals to be taken. Medications to be given out. Liz took a medication to relax her before her surgery, and she was wheeled from the room half asleep.

Dr. Harris came into the room, calling for a nurse to help him remove my dressings. He gloved up, then carefully and gently removed layer after layer.

I glanced at all the familiar parts of my body, assuring myself that I was prepared for what would come next. This is the acid test, I thought.

"There," he said. "Looks pretty good—not too much swelling. Actually, I'm surprised. Considering the amount of surgery we did, I would have expected more."

At first, I couldn't make myself look down at the incision. Then I instructed myself: You have to do this. Look down now.

The first glance was shocking. I felt strangely disoriented, but I couldn't stop looking. It was like staring at something that was not part of my body. A long diagonal scar ran from the centre of my chest to somewhere underneath my arm. I thought of a railroad track crossing a prairie.

I was aware of a deep sadness. I felt suspended, poised in a love-hate relationship with the asymmetry of my physical being. Perhaps the morphine contributed to the disorientation; many of my experiences in the hospital had seemed fragmented or dreamlike. I remembered how the doctor had said he'd removed everything that wasn't nailed down. To me it looked like a war zone—they may have saved the country but, my God, look what they did to the land.

"Take a deep breath for a minute," Dr. Harris suggested. "I'm going to remove this drainage tube."

I closed my eyes, holding my breath. I felt nothing as he

pulled out the long tube with one quick tug. He firmly palpated the skin around the incision. Although there was a sense of pressure, I couldn't feel his fingers on my skin. I watched as he started to cover the area with a new, clean dressing.

"It's a shock, isn't it," he said softly, looking at my face. "But time is a great healer."

I felt a terrible coldness. I wondered if I would ever be warm again. My mind was racing. I knew I should feel lucky. Despite its large size, Dr. Harris had said the tumour had been contained. I took this to mean that it hadn't grown beyond the breast itself, and I tried to hold on to that thought. I made every effort to stay optimistic about the lab results I would soon receive.

"I think we can get rid of this intravenous now," he said, removing the catheter and pressing on the insertion site. He waited until the nurse handed him a new dressing. "But I should mention that you lost a lot of blood during the surgery. Considering that the first surgery wasn't long ago, I'd suggest you get yourself onto some iron pills when you get home. We could have given you a blood transfusion, but we don't do that unless it's absolutely necessary."

He picked up my frog and raised his eyebrows in question.

"A cancer-cell eater," I explained.

"Aah, of course." He nodded approvingly, handing the frog back to me. "We had better start cutting the morphine back, but we won't do that today—you're probably going to be pretty sore after what I've just done."

He gave my foot a squeeze. "I'll see you tomorrow," he said.

I felt very restless. My mind had slipped into over-drive. I got out of bed and put on my bathrobe. I stood at the window, looking down towards a grassy area with trees I hadn't noticed before. They looked as though someone had hacked them with an axe; the limbs were deformed and grotesque. I remembered some words from a poem I had once written: *If you don't think about it, perhaps it won't have happened. If you don't say it, perhaps it won't be true.*

I decided I needed a walk. I allowed my hand to slip inside my robe, gently exploring the new geography of my body. Nausea rose sudden as fear. I bustled past the nurses' station to a visitors' bathroom, made sure the door was locked and braced myself over the sink while the walls moved around me. I thought about how often I had responded to calls for "a collapse in the bathroom," and how people instinctively flee or hide when they fear they are losing it. I was no exception.

There was a humming in my ears, and I was in such a cold sweat that I was dripping onto one of my hands. I sat on the toilet and put my head between my knees. I couldn't think for the life of me what I had learned about fainting in my training as a paramedic. I could only remember what I had been taught as a child. I stayed in that position until the floor and walls no longer swirled.

Eventually, I leaned my head back against the wall. Something terrible had been done to me, and I had felt both helpless to prevent it and helpless in the face of it. Like a head-on collision, I thought. I was like someone who can only ask, "What happened, what happened?"

I wiped the perspiration off my forehead, noticing that my skin was only wet on the left side of my face. I stood up and slowly made my way back to the ward.

I slept off and on for the rest of the morning. Between dozes, I was aware that Liz Berry had been brought back from surgery, and I heard Jessie talking with someone. Mississippi was finally moved to palliative care. As she was wheeled out of the room, I heard Jessie sigh, "Thank God."

Liz Berry, still under the effects of the anaesthetic, slept soundly. A nurse tiptoed in and took her vitals.

But moments after the nurse left, I heard Liz gagging. I pushed myself off the side of the bed. "Nurse," I shouted through the open door.

A nurse marched into the room. "What's all the fussing about?"

"Quick, she's vomiting."

The nurse rolled Liz onto her side, shouting for assistance. I stepped back and let a swarm of nurses take over. One of them asked, "Do you think she aspirated—"

"I don't know," I said before she had even finished her question. "I got to her right away, but she had already thrown up." I looked at my right arm, which hung uselessly against my side. "I couldn't roll her—"

"Watch your step," someone else warned, pointing to the floor. "We'll ring for an orderly to clean up the mess."

Liz's bed was pushed out the door. No doubt she was headed for the intensive care unit. I washed my hands, changed my gown and climbed gratefully into my bed. But I couldn't stop thinking of her. If only I'd had the use of my right arm, but my shoulder had refused to budge. I was surprised, because I had thought it was simply pain that had kept me from using it.

I hadn't been back in bed for long when several of my friends dropped by for a visit. I watched Pat as she tended to my flowers. She shook out the wet stems, stripped the lower leaves, snapped off the ends and put the flowers back in the water. It was soothing to watch her. There weren't enough chairs, so some people sat on the edge of the bed. I knew I was in trouble. They soon had me laughing so hard that I was perspiring from the pain. The more they fussed over keeping me from laughing, the more I laughed.

Another friend arrived just as everyone had stood up to leave. She handed me a plant, which I couldn't hold on to. It hit the floor with a thunderous crash.

We all stared in amazement. A bottle of Kahlúa had been hidden beneath the greenery. The plant and the bottle were in pieces on the floor. The smell of alcohol slowly filled the ward.

My friend shrugged. "Sorry," she said. "It seemed like a good idea."

A nurse burst into the room. "What is going on?" she demanded, slowly taking in the scene.

"Just a little accident." I smiled apologetically, but the nurse smiled not at all.

"Well, I suppose I'll have to call the orderly again," she complained.

Pat suggested they all leave. "I think we've done this old thing in," she said.

It was the same orderly who had cleaned the floor earlier. "What is it about this room?" he asked. I smiled as if it had nothing to do with me. I fell asleep to the sound of his mop swishing back and forth.

When I woke, I realized from the light outside the window that I must have been asleep for hours. Katherine was sitting in the chair beside the bed. "Hi, Mozer."

"Hi, darling, how long have you been here?"

"Not too long. I hope I didn't wake you up." She leaned over the bed and gave me a kiss.

As she sat back down, Dr. Harris walked into the room. I was surprised. I hadn't expected to see him again until the next day.

I looked at Katherine. "Would you mind leaving us for a minute?"

Dr. Harris seemed to hesitate a long time before he said anything. I braced myself.

"I've mentioned to you that when we did your surgery, your lymph nodes were enlarged—that is why we removed so many. I've been quite concerned, so I went to the lab myself this afternoon." He smiled. "Good news—the lymph nodes are clear."

Say something, I told myself, but it was as if a kind of paralysis had hit me. What was he saying? Did this mean I had a better chance of staying alive? Did it mean I wouldn't need radiation and chemotherapy?

"I'm delightfully surprised," he added. "From the size of the tumour I had feared bad news. You must have high host resistance, or the cancer would certainly have metastasized throughout your body."

He patted my foot through the blankets. "Anyway, I wanted you to know right away. We'll see how you're doing tomorrow. Perhaps you can go home." He smiled. And then he was gone.

Katherine came back into the room. Apprehension showed in her eyes, the set of her face.

"It's not in the nodes," I said quickly. She wrapped her arms around me. "I didn't even thank him," I said. She sat on the side of my bed, holding my hand. We grinned at each other for a long time.

Eventually, I walked her to the elevators. Then I paced back and forth through the halls, trying to understand what this new information meant to me. As I rounded a corner, I stopped. Like a mirage, Deirdre came into view.

We gave each other a long hug. I felt a happiness, warm and flooding. "God, it's so good to see you," I said.

"I can't believe it," she said through watery eyes. "I just can't believe it. I had this vision of you lying in bed looking half-dead with tubes all over the place."

Like her father, I thought. I was happy to let her know my good news.

"But didn't I tell you?" She gave me another long hug. "I've thought of you so often."

She followed me into the room. I was shocked to see that beneath her newly acquired tan, she still looked exhausted. I dragged a chair close to the bed with my foot. "How come you've been away and you still look tired?"

"It was a long trip home."

"Everything else is okay?"

"Everything's fine."

We talked about her trip until the dinner trays arrived. She rose and walked around the bed touching this and that flower, talking. I closed my eyes, content to float on her words.

"Do you know what the best part of the whole trip was?" I could tell she had stopped moving about. I opened my eyes. She was smiling down at me.

"You may not believe this, but I went to church. It was one of my most beautiful moments on this earth: birds singing—"

"An outdoor service?"

She nodded. "Hawaiian families—dressed as colourfully as these flowers—danced to the Lord's Prayer. Now you tell me, when was the last time you danced to the Lord's Prayer?"

I started to laugh. In a corner of my mind, I imagined her amidst the lush tropical greenery and flowers. It seemed right.

"I thought of you a lot during that service," she said. "I kind of felt I was with you."

We stared at each other. Her dark eyes were soft, deeper somehow. She placed her hand, gently clinking with bracelets, on top of mine. I felt her touch somewhere deep inside. I became aware of my heart. There was no pain, no irregularity in its rhythm. I was merely aware of its boundless, undeniable beating.

Suddenly, she pushed the table with my dinner in close to me. "Eat," she said. "You need to get well enough so you can spring out of this place and get better."

I told her I hoped to be home the next day. We drifted back into our old routine of easy banter. She talked, while I braved a few bites of the dinner.

"It's not exactly Peter's elegant cooking, is it?" she said, noticing how slowly the food made it to my mouth.

I sighed. "I think they've reheated breakfast."

"I'll drop by and see you at home tomorrow," she said, slipping her jacket on. She squeezed her eyes shut and made the motions of imaginary paddling. "In the summer," she said. "You and me. It won't be long."

I had packed everything, and I was ready to leave. My clothes felt strangely restrictive, but they also made me feel I had achieved some outward likeness of recovery.

A student nurse bounced into the room with a little paper cup containing two blue pills. "What are they?" I asked.

"They're 292s—codeine to help you with any discomfort on your way home."

I looked at the pills again. If these were 292s, I was Florence Nightingale.

"Would you check these pills? These are not 292s."

I could tell she wasn't sure what to do, but she withdrew from the room with the pills in hand.

"By the way," I called after her, "if they're something really good, please bring them back."

"They trying to poison you or something?" Jessie asked.

"I think so. Surgery didn't do me in, so they're taking one last stab, so to speak."

Jessie laughed so hard her whole bed shook.

"So your big surgery is tomorrow?" I asked.

"You got it—tomorrow I'm on an instant weight reduction plan." She cupped her large hand under her breast. "I figure this thing must be a few pounds."

It was my turn to laugh. "Good for you," I said.

The student nurse came back timidly with two familiar-looking pills. "I'm really curious," I said, swallowing them. "What were the blue ones?"

She gave me an uncertain smile and disappeared. For a moment or two, perhaps cancer had been the least of my worries.

The nurse had left a sheet of paper with instructions on how to live with no nodes on one side. The list seemed so amusing to me that I read it out loud to Jessie, adding a few cautions of my own: "I am not to have my blood pressure taken on my right side. I am not to get shots or sunburns on my right arm—no mosquito bites, no hangnails, no cuts, burns or pimples. I am to wear a thimble while sewing and gloves while washing dishes or gardening. I am not to wear tight jewellery or tight sleeves."

Jessie and I entertained ourselves until a woman I didn't know walked into the room. "Hi, I'm Jane, from Reach to Recovery," she introduced herself. "Ten years ago, I went through what you're going through now. May I take a minute or two of your time?"

I remained silent, but nodded.

"Do you know about Reach to Recovery?"

"I've heard about it."

"Our group was started by a woman named Terese Lasser, who had a mastectomy in 1952. Her surgery and cancer caused her to go into a deep depression. After she pulled herself out of it, she decided to form a support group to help other women."

Jane paused for a moment and looked at everything stacked on my bed. "Is there anything you need? Any questions you might have?"

"Please, sit down," I said, finally.

"You're just on your way home?" She smiled, easing herself into a chair.

"Yes, my husband will be arriving shortly."

She handed me a nondescript plastic bag. I looked inside. It was full of what looked like stuffing.

"It's very soft," she explained. "You won't want a prosthesis for a while, until you are nicely healed. So when your bandages come off, you can just pin some of this stuffing into the cup of your bra and it won't irritate the incision."

I could feel the colour rise in my cheeks. For some reason, I hadn't thought that far ahead. I had no idea what a breast prosthesis looked like, or how it was worn, or whether or not I wanted one. I had seen amputees with an artificial arm or leg, but surprisingly, never a breast. I knew this was the woman to ask, but I simply didn't have the nerve.

"You said ten years ago?" I asked, to make conversation.

"Ten years ago tomorrow."

"You haven't had a recurrence?"

"No. I've been doing really well."

Peter walked into the room. I introduced him to Jane. "She had the surgery ten years ago," I explained.

He smiled broadly but was quiet. Jane excused herself and left me her name and phone number. "Call any time," she said.

I put her card and number into my pocket.

Peter looked anxious. He was staring at all the flowers and gifts I had accumulated.

"Don't panic," I said. "Most of these flowers are staying. Those are going upstairs to Mississippi's room; those over there are for the nurses' station, and one of the nurses is checking to see what room Liz Berry is in."

"Mrs. MacPhee," a nurse called from the doorway. "I checked on the computer, and there isn't a patient by the name of Liz Berry."

I was stunned. I figured Liz would have made it out of intensive care by now. I glanced at the nurse. But I didn't ask. I was handling all I could for the moment.

Peter made several trips down to the car and then arrived with a wheelchair for me. "No arguing," he warned, but I was far from wanting to argue. My legs were rubbery. I was moving with one breast from the security of the hospital into the world of the normal.

The cool afternoon air hit me with a shock. Peter opened the car door and helped me into the seat. He was treating me like glass. He even drove as if I were made of glass. But it was true that I felt every bump.

I looked out the car window at all the familiar streets. My protective wall had begun to crumble. It was not me riding in this car but someone else, and I was watching—watching a woman whose hands were shaking. I felt better when I closed my eyes, and I did so for several miles. I didn't open them until Peter geared down to climb the long curving road up the mountain.

10

AS WE PULLED INTO our driveway, I felt scared. This was home. I wanted to give my family a sense of normality. But I wasn't sure I could be what I thought they expected and needed me to be.

Katherine and Jenny ran down the stairs to greet me. Katherine handed me a pillow to hold against my front so that Freyja, in the excitement of welcoming me, would do no damage.

I hadn't been home for more than a few minutes before I felt the need to go to bed. I loved our bed. But I could see it was going to be a little more challenging now to get in and out of.

I lay down, wrapped in the protective walls of the house. There wasn't a sound. Everyone was so quiet I wondered what they could possibly be doing. I tried to comfort myself that they had all gone out for a walk. And then I knew. They were doing nothing so that they wouldn't disturb me.

I heard a sound. It took me a moment to realize that it had come from me. I had cried out.

Peter stood beside the bed. "Are you okay?"

"I just had a horrible dream."

"Can you remember it?"

"I could a second ago, but now it's gone."

"Can I get you anything?"

"Perhaps some tea." I rolled onto my left side, making the swimming motions of trying to get up.

"I'm happy to bring it to you," Peter said, offering me a hand.

"No—I'd like to get up."

I made my way downstairs. Peter and Jenny finished bringing everything in from the car while Katherine made the tea.

"What have all of you been doing while I was sleeping?" I asked Katherine. "The house was so quiet."

"Jenny and I took Freyja to the waterfall, and I think Dad was reading downstairs."

"You know, I'm used to the noise of the hospital. Please don't feel you have to tiptoe around. A little noise and confusion is better for me right now than silence."

Katherine gave me a gentle hug. "It's sure nice to have you home, Mozer."

"Thank you, darling. It's good to be home."

I sat at the dining room table looking out at the sky. There was a scattering of dark angry clouds. As I sat and drank my tea, I watched the sky darken. The green of the trees and mountains darkened too.

I looked around the house. It seemed to be full of broken things: a chair to be repaired, cracked pottery, a twisted lampshade. Beside me, the needle in the barometer was swinging to *Low*. Peter had taped a cardboard silhouette of a hawk to one of the windows, trying to deter small birds from flying into the glass. Apart from the hawk, everything looked normal. Everything looked the same. That should have comforted me, but it didn't. I no longer felt the same. I thought of Jessie saying, "You just want the thing off so everything can get back to the way it was." But it didn't seem to work like that. I had no idea how anything could ever again be the way it was. I was home. I was supposed to be all right now. But I didn't feel all right. I felt as weak and wobbly as a baby.

Jenny handed me a card that Pat had sent. She had written her phone number at the bottom, as if I might have forgotten it. Between the lines of her message, I read, I don't want to disturb you. Call me.

The dream I'd had was so vivid it affected the rest of my day. I felt irritated, annoyed. But no matter how hard I tried to remember the dream, it floated just out of reach.

Peter prepared a delicious dinner. He offered me wine or beer. I decided on a beer, but my stomach told me immediately that it had been a mistake.

My right breast was hurting more now than it had in the hospital. Since the surgery, I'd had a lot of stabbing pains that seemed to start nowhere and end nowhere. Sometimes there were electrical sensations like nerves firing. Other times the pains were sharp enough to take my breath away. But tonight was different somehow. There was a terrible numbness in my right breast that I hadn't felt before.

You don't have a right breast, I reminded myself.

"Do you want me to sleep downstairs tonight?" Peter asked. "I don't want to roll into you in the night."

"No, I'll be fine," I said, wondering briefly if he'd asked because he'd prefer to sleep by himself. But I wanted him close.

The problem for me would be finding a comfortable way to sleep. I couldn't lie on my stomach or my right side. When I was on my left side, the weight of my right arm against my body was a problem. As for lying on my back, it made me feel like a stiff laid out in the morgue.

Standing before the mirror in the dark of the bedroom, the person I saw didn't look different from the person I remembered. I thought, I am the same and not the same. The area of my body that was missing didn't really show. But somehow the numbness I felt was even worse than the pain, because the numbness meant that part of my body was dead.

I climbed into a loose pair of Peter's pyjamas and slipped under the quilt. I was exhausted. When Peter came to bed, he held me gently and at a distance. We fell asleep to the sound of rain.

I woke with a start. The dream had returned. The harder I tried to focus on it, the more elusive it seemed. It was so real that I was afraid to sleep. I listened to the rain until it eased off. I couldn't wait for the night to be over.

Eventually I must have dropped off, because I woke up to music. I was relieved that the clock-radio had switched itself on. Listening to the newscast, I was surprised that the world was still talking about the war in Kuwait. The war was over and, to me, it seemed to have happened so long ago.

A Tornado squadron leader who had just returned from the Gulf was introduced as one of America's most experienced pilots, flying fighter-bombers for eighteen years. "After two of our Tornadoes were lost, I cried," he said proudly. "I shed more tears in those last forty days than in my last forty years." I thought of Shannon, Liz, Jessie and Mississippi, and all the other women I had seen pacing the halls of the hospital.

Peter was in the shower. I looked for something to wear, then decided I was as comfortable as I could be in his baggy pyjamas. I got unsteadily to my feet. The rain had almost stopped, and the ocean was a vague shimmer of dull light. I felt listless and strange.

Peter joined me in the dining room. Dressed in a dark suit, he looked strong and solid. I stood up and adjusted his tie with my left hand.

"What can I get for you?" he asked, kissing my cheek gently.

"A cup of coffee might be a good jump-start."

"Some breakfast?"

"No, thanks," I said. "I'll make myself something."

"Then I'll be off." He gave me a kiss and called from the door, "I'll phone before I come home in case you want me to pick up anything."

Jenny came running up the stairs and rushed past me, grabbing a banana from the kitchen. On her way back out, she stopped and we gave each other a quick hug. "I love you," she said.

"I love you too. And the banana breakfast!" I shouted. "Let me get you something else."

"Haven't time, Mom. Bye." The door slammed shut.

I sat for a while at the table. On the deck below, a few birds pecked at scattered seeds. I looked at my watch. Only five minutes had gone by. It would be a long day.

I felt cold. I put on my robe and walked to my desk. I sat listening to the quiet.

"What are you up to, Mozer?" Katherine asked, suddenly appearing from nowhere.

I stared at her blankly, caught myself, and said, "A bath— I've been thinking how nice it would be to have a bath. Would you help me wash my hair?"

"Sure."

I would have much preferred a shower, but I had to keep my dressings dry. While Katherine ran the water, I tried to think of some way to do this without removing my pyjamas. I hadn't felt self-conscious in the hospital because the doctors and nurses were used to the sight of lopsided bodies. In that environment, I was normal; here I wasn't. Yet I knew Katherine should get used to seeing me with the dressings. Then perhaps the sight of my body without the packaging wouldn't be such a shock. My stomach tightened at the thought that my body might shock someone.

She sat beside the tub while I carefully washed myself. I heard her say, "What has happened to you—" Her voice broke off. "It's not fair—you didn't deserve this."

"Well, I don't know that it has anything to do with what's fair or what you deserve," I answered as brightly as possible. "Not really. It's just the way it is."

My response wasn't much of an answer, but it was all I had to offer.

Her eyes remained fixed on me. Eventually she asked, "How are we going to do your hair?"

"Probably easiest if I just lean over the sink. Does that sound workable to you?"

"No problem. Here, let me help dry you."

She did so very gently. I was reminded of all the times—not so long ago—when she was little and I'd be drying her off. I wrapped a towel around myself, spa style, and found that with one breast the towel didn't stay up easily. I had to hold it in place while Katherine washed my hair. I put on my robe as she towel-dried my head.

When I was dressed I went back downstairs. Katherine had put the mail on the dining room table. The first thing I saw was another card from Pat. Inside, she had written: "I can't stop cleaning—please get better quickly—I don't want to clean. Tu amiga, Patricia."

There was also a postcard from an old friend, Elaine. Elaine had been in Europe touring art galleries for several months. I recognized the picture on the front of the postcard right away; it was Picasso's *Woman Asleep in a Red Armchair*. Only one of the woman's breasts was visible, and her hands were held on her lap in such a way that they hid her genitals. Elaine had written: "Dearest Roz: Found this card the other day and although I'm not sure why, it made me think of you. Maybe it's because if you were here you'd laugh if you saw all the boobs. Picasso, in particular, had a penchant for women with an irregular number. Take care of yourself. With love, Elaine."

I read the card again. How bizarre, I thought to myself. Katherine peeled me an orange and poured some coffee. "I'll let you have some honey in your coffee if you tell me what you're thinking about." She held the honey jar just out of my reach. "You look far away."

"Here, read this card from Elaine and tell me what you think. She's been in Europe for months. She doesn't know I have breast cancer or that I've had surgery."

Katherine read silently, then smiled. "What I think is that we don't know the first thing about life. I think that on some level she does know." She handed the card back to me. "It's kind of strange, isn't it? Particularly because you've been studying Picasso."

"It's weird."

Katherine went into the kitchen to pour herself another coffee. "Have you figured out what you're going to do about your course?"

"There is no way I can write my final exam next week. I don't seem to be able to remember what I've read by the time I get to the end of a card."

"Ask your doctor for a letter. I'm sure the university would let you do the exam at a later date."

"Maybe, but—" I saw the challenge in her eyes. I returned the look, then gave in. "Well, I just might try the letter idea. Somehow I had figured I'd have the surgery and life would be back to normal." I raised my eyebrows at her. "It's not exactly working out that way, is it?"

"You expect so much from yourself."

I decided to ignore her comment. "Speaking of university, don't *you* still have exams you should be studying for?"

She didn't answer right away. I looked at her as she played with the orange peel. "I've withdrawn from university," she said, meeting my eyes.

"But why?" I asked. "It's not because of me, is it?"

"No," she said. "Not really. I admit I've been worried about you, and that has made it harder to study. But I lost interest a long time ago. University is just not what I want."

"You're almost finished your second year."

"Mom, I wouldn't have passed the exams."

"But you've always done so well."

"That was when I thought university was where I wanted to be."

I closed my eyes. "I appreciate having you at home so much," I said. "I honestly don't know how I'd be coping if I were on my own—but not at the cost of sabotaging your university."

"And you're not! I'll get really angry if you can't accept that. I didn't want to tell you this right now, but I also didn't want to lie to you. I'm not ashamed of having withdrawn. I believe it's the right thing for me to do."

We looked at each other silently for a moment. "Mom, you've always said that nobody can teach you about life."

I smiled. "Actually, that's an expression borrowed from Pat."

"Well, you believe it, don't you?"

"Absolutely."

"So relax. Everything is okay. Right?"

"Right," I repeated. "Everything's okay."

"Here, let me get you a fresh cup of coffee. You haven't touched yours."

When I finally lay down for a rest, I went over our conversation from as many angles as I could. Although I wanted to be totally supportive of whatever Katherine did, I was disappointed. She was a thinker, and I couldn't see her being happy unless she had access to a lot of ideas. Universities were good for that. I felt guilty about having caused this interruption in her education.

I remembered something Pat had said just after the slide. "You know, Roz, people get these big challenges in their lives and somehow they cope with them." She had pointed to some sofa cushions that had been soiled by their cat during an attack of diarrhea. "It's all the other shit that doesn't stop that does you in."

We had laughed together then, and I smiled now.

I slept for most of the day; got up for dinner, ate, looked at my watch and went back to bed.

I woke in the night. I was out of breath and soaked in perspiration. Peter was holding me. "You're okay," he said. "You're okay. You've been screaming, 'Run.' Tell me what you've been dreaming."

I closed my eyes and tried to concentrate on slowing my breathing. "I'm all right now," I said.

Peter held me until finally I fell back into a fitful sleep: *I will save no lives, I realize; everyone is too far gone. Some, with deformed heads and bodies, look as if they have been hacked about with an axe, and yet there is no blood. Everything is strangely monochromatic: light reflects from the angular surfaces, one head like a wedge of bone, another misshapen like a dog's, another face stony, masklike. With some, their backs and faces are both visible at the same time. It is impossible to understand how they are able to move at all with those slow swimming motions, but I can see the rise and fall of light, of limbs at strange angles, while other limbs merge almost completely with each other. And then I see movement. A blue shadow moving randomly, and without sound, hacking the bodies into chunks, striking again and again. I see my daughters, and I whisper to them, Run. But they don't run. I don't understand. Why don't they run? I scream at my daughters, Run. But it is only my own legs running, my own mouth screaming, screaming without sound ...*

In my sleep, I had rolled onto my right side, and I woke from the pain. Peter was already up. The bedroom window was high with mountains and sky. Blue sky. For the first time since I'd been home, I could tell the hour by the sun's position over the mountain.

I had an appointment with Dr. Harris that morning, and my first challenge was to decide what to wear. I made my way through shirts, sweaters and jackets. I rummaged in a drawer until I found my loosest sports bra, and the bra extensor I'd had since I was pregnant with Jenny. A lot of extra fluid had accumulated in the tissue around my incision—lympho-edema. I wasn't sure I'd be able to wear a bra, but with the extensor piece it was reasonably comfortable.

I studied the empty right cup. What to do with it? At the moment, the pressure dressings took up part of the space, but I would probably be coming home with a flat dressing. I stuffed in some nylon stockings, but I didn't have enough. The shoul-der pads from a silk blouse didn't work either, because they rubbed. I picked up a handful of the stuffing the woman from Reach to Recovery had given me. Determinedly, I shoved it crudely into the cup. But it had no weight. Even though I didn't look off-kilter, I certainly felt that way—one wrong move and one breast would be higher or lower than the other. I eyed a drawer full of Peter's socks.

"Not bad," I said out loud as I looked at my new curves in the mirror. I fell back into a chair, soaked with sweat. All these decisions had worn me out. "Don't despair," I said to my reflection. "Remember that you come from a long line of professional soldiers." I knew that I shared two qualities with these ancestral leaders: the ability to push on, and luck.

I remembered the conversation with my sister in St. Louis when I'd called to tell her about the breast cancer. "My God, what a lot happens to you," she'd said. I didn't respond, but I gave it some thought. When she phoned after the surgery to see how I was doing, she said, "Well, no matter what you fall into, you always seem to come up smelling like a rose." Her parting words were, "Remember, nothing gets a Roberts girl down."

"Wrong," I said out loud.

"Did you call, Mozer?" Katherine asked from the kitchen.

"Nope—just talking to myself."

The perspiring had eased off, but I felt damp. I noticed that I was still not perspiring on the right side of my face and upper body.

I left the socks in the right cup of my bra and got on with dressing. Casual clothing was what this situation called for, and lots of it. I dressed in a denim outfit that made me feel the most like me, and then I threw on a jacket. "It's the layered look," I mumbled, assessing the total picture in the mirror. Deirdre would probably say that at long last I was in style.

Outside the protective shelter of my house, I felt nervous. Katherine sat beside me in the waiting room. I looked around at the other faces and realized that mine was probably the most relaxed one there. For the first time, I had a sense of moving through the process. I closed my eyes and went over all the questions I wanted to ask the doctor.

Before long I was in the examination room. Once I'd exchanged my clothes for a gown, I felt very cold. Using my left hand, I tried to throw my jacket around my shoulders, but after it fell on the floor twice, I gave up and moved to a chair by the window, where there was a heater. As I waited for the door to open, my anxiety level hit a new high. I worked at convincing myself that this was a conditioned response brought about by my previous experiences here.

When Dr. Harris finally appeared, we made some small talk about how "fine" I felt and then he said, "So, let's have a look."

He loosened the edges of the bandages and gave me a sidelong glance. "Think tough for a second. I'm just going to give this dressing a little tug—and there we have it."

I looked down at where my breast used to be. The skin was very tight, and the edges of the incision looked thick and red and angry.

Dr. Harris kept his eyes on my face as his hands pressed gently but firmly all over my chest. My God, I thought, he is looking for a lump that got away. I could feel my blood shunting away from my extremities to my vital organs as if I were a container of fluid that had been tipped the wrong way.

"Are you okay?"

I nodded, but I knew I was in trouble.

"Let's lie you down for a minute," he said, helping me onto the examination table. "Better?"

"Yes."

He pulled a chair up beside me and sat down. "How's it going at home?" he asked.

"Good. But I'm always cold. I feel very weak and—weepy. I don't cry," I was quick to point out. "It's just that the tears are really close to the surface."

"You feel that way because you've lost a lot of blood," he explained. "Don't forget you've had two surgeries in a very short period of time. It's only ten days since your mastectomy. Sometimes there is a residual effect from the anaesthetics, too." He folded his arms over his chest. "We'll do some more blood tests. I wouldn't be surprised if you're anaemic. In the hospital I suggested you take an iron supplement—"

I nodded. "I have been."

"Good. Go easy on yourself. You've been through an amputation as well as dealing with something that is life-threatening."

"What about the pain? How long until ..."

"It's different for every woman. For most women it eases off in a few months. But for some women it's a year or two. For others—" He paused for a moment and then explained, "Nerve endings are very sensitive. It's usually easier after the skin stretches." He put his hands behind his head and tipped back a little in his chair. "You know you have done extremely well, don't you?"

I nodded.

"Duncan and I were talking about you the other day. You've handled all of this so well. We've decided that your paramedic training to deal with emergencies must have helped you through this."

He let his chair settle back on all four legs. Then he pulled a tissue out of a box and handed it to me.

"Feeling better?" he asked.

"Yes."

"Okay. I'm going to remove these stitches and then cover the incision to protect it from infection."

He placed the box of tissues beside me and went to work. "Keep in mind that you don't have those infection-fighting lymph nodes under your right arm any more, so we want to keep this area as sterile as we can while it is healing."

"Can you talk while you work?" I asked.

"Something you're wondering about?"

"What is your guess as to how long I've had breast cancer?"

"Well, judging from the size of the lump—probably more than eight years."

"Eight years," I said loudly. "I've had breast cancer for eight years and I haven't even known it?"

He nodded. "At least eight, I'd think. That's not uncommon. Breast cancers tend to be sneaky. They aren't feelable until they are a pretty good size. And yours was pretty deep."

"I guess if I had been checking my breasts, I would have found it sooner—perhaps increased my chances of survival?"

"Breast cancer is not all good management. The majority of women who come in here have found their lump while in the shower, or rolling over in bed. Or a husband or a lover finds it."

He applied a thin layer of dressing and then stepped back to assess his work. "But we are going to get all this behind you. Right?"

"Right," I answered, forcing a smile.

He felt down my right arm and turned the palm of my hand towards him. "The swelling really isn't bad. I think we can get you started on some nice gentle exercise." He walked over to the wall. "What I want you to do is just what you see me doing. Walk your fingers up the wall like so, slowly … just until it starts to hurt. It's important not to force your arm, or you will have no end of problems with swelling. If the swelling gets too bad I can draw off some of the fluid with a needle. But that's not necessary at the moment. Let's see you do it."

I slipped off the examination table and extended my arm towards the wall in front of me. Although it was discouraging to see that my fingers would not climb higher than waist level, I felt relieved to be given something to do to help things along.

"Fine," he said. "Twice a day. And do what I'm doing right now. Just dangle your arm loosely at your side and then start moving it around in small circles, letting the circles get bigger and bigger as your body is willing."

I watched what he was doing and then followed his motions.

He nodded approvingly as he watched my feeble efforts. "That's to keep your shoulder from freezing up on you."

I smiled. "I think I can handle this."

"Here is a requisition for some blood work. How's the pain medication holding out?"

"Almost gone," I answered.

He handed me a prescription. "Remember—don't push that arm. It's been severely traumatized, and it's going to need time to heal. And patience. Some women end up needing more surgery to fix up the damage they do to themselves. When you're ready, I'll send you to a physiotherapist. Then you can work on getting back your range of motion."

"When do you think I can return to work?"

He studied me carefully. "For the kind of work you do, I think you're looking at about two months from the date of surgery."

"That's more than six weeks from now," I protested. "You said I'd be off for a month."

"Yes. But that was taking things one step at a time. You've had extensive surgery and you have a physically demanding job. What's important is that you *are* going to get there." He looked at me for a moment as if allowing time for his words to sink in. "As you know, the lab tests confirmed the nodes were clear. Negative nodes indicate that chemotherapy is not needed, but it's often given for large tumours these days. Because of the size of your tumour, chemotherapy might not be a bad idea. I've discussed your case with Dr. Thompson. He's an oncologist. He doesn't feel you need that treatment unless it's your wish. I'd be happy to refer you to him."

"You said the lymph nodes were enlarged when you did the surgery."

"Yes, they were. That's why I was pretty aggressive with the surgery—and also because the tumour was large."

"Why do you think the nodes were enlarged?"

He shrugged his shoulders. "Hard to say. Perhaps your body was fighting off some kind of infection at the time. Or it's possible that your lymph system may have been active in response to the cancer."

"Maybe it was the Mexican food." I smiled. "One of my friends was frightened I'd get Montezuma's revenge and not be able to have the surgery."

"Well, all in all, things have worked out pretty well," he said, sounding pleased. "With that tan of yours you were the healthiest-looking patient in the hospital. Do you want to think about the chemotherapy?"

"No. I've already made that decision. I decided that unless you told me I was going to die in an hour or two without it, I would say thanks, but no thanks."

"If you change your mind, or if you want to talk to Dr. Thompson yourself, just let me know."

"Okay, but I don't think I'll change my mind. I've dreaded the chemotherapy. I couldn't bear to feel any weaker than I already do. I don't want to feel sick all the time and throw up everything I eat. I'm having a hard enough time as it is." I looked him directly in the eye. "I don't want it for myself or for my family and friends."

"It's not that bad for everyone."

"I've seen it. People get sick on chemotherapy. It makes them susceptible to infection, and some people even die from the complications. The books don't tend to inform you about a lot of that."

"That's extreme. And if you need the treatment, it is the least of the evils," he reminded me, standing up to wash his hands. "If a woman has lymph node involvement, she has a much greater chance of adding some years to her life with chemotherapy."

"I can't tell you how relieved I am that I don't have to have it."

He glanced over towards the window. My clothing had fallen off the back of the chair, and there on the floor lay my bra and Peter's socks, looking like skeins of wool flowing over the rim of a basket. I felt my blood flow full-force back to my cheeks.

Dr. Harris smiled. "In about a month, we'll send you to be fitted for a prosthesis. That will make you feel better. We have to wait for enough healing before you wear one. In the meantime, if you like, you could get a soft foam prosthesis. They only cost a few dollars. There's a place just down the road where you can pick one up and get your prescription filled at the same time."

There was that word again. "When do you want to see me next?" I asked, pulling my clothes onto my lap.

"In about a week." He paused. "Would you like some assistance getting dressed?"

"No, thank you." I smiled at him. "I have a system."

"See you next week then," he said.

As I walked into the waiting room, I glanced at the faces and said a silent prayer for each woman: May you be surrounded with love.

"How did it go?" Katherine asked when we were out in the hall.

"Well," I answered, waving my prescription and the requisition for blood work in the air.

The lab did my blood test right away. The technician gently massaged some of my bruised veins and commented, "Looks like you've had a few of these recently."

"Please don't take any more blood than you need," I said. "Mine is a little thin these days."

When I was finished, Katherine and I headed for the pharmacy. She walked beside me with her hand protectively on my arm. "So what did he say?"

"I'm supposed to buy a ... a pro-sthes-is."

"I hadn't even thought of that," Katherine said. "I tend to think of a prosthesis as a false arm or leg."

"Me too. At least you can say the word." I repeated it softly several times, trying to perfect its pronunciation, while Katherine laughed at me.

"God, I might as well give up. I have enough trouble saying mast-ec-to-my. I used to be able to say it as part of my job, but as soon as I heard I had to have one, I could no longer produce the right sounds."

Katherine grinned. "I wonder what a linguist would say about that."

"It may be called a mental block."

We stopped outside the pharmacy. I took a deep breath and said, "Here goes."

I looked after the prescription first. It was for a hundred pills; Dr. Harris was obviously expecting me to need pain medication for a while.

As the pharmacist filled the prescription, I noticed a small, discreet sign that read "Breast Prostheses." Foam breasts in graduated sizes covered the wall. They were wrapped neatly in transparent plastic packages. I decided that these must be the temporary prostheses the doctor had mentioned. I selected one that looked the right size for me. It felt almost as if it were full of air.

A rack of bathing suits stood next to the wall of prostheses. They looked surprisingly normal, but came up higher than a regular suit under the arms and at the neck. They had special pockets where you could slip in your prosthesis, right or left. It occurred to me that some women had to slip in a right *and* a left. The thought gave me the willies.

Then I saw the real thing sitting in a little display that had been made specially for it. I picked it up. It was heavy, like a breast. It even had something that resembled a nipple. It felt cold, but as I held it, I realized it was absorbing the warmth of my hand. I gave it a squeeze. It felt like a breast. As I settled it back in its display cradle, its outer surface wrinkled.

"May I help you?" A woman had come up beside me.

"Not at the moment," I said uneasily. "I've just had surgery. I understand I need to wait about a month before wearing one of these."

She nodded. "In the meantime, you might like to use the kind you have in your hand. They hand-wash nicely," she said. "I wouldn't suggest you put them in the dryer—they can get lumpy."

She handed me a brochure, pointing to the real prostheses. "These are wonderful," she said. "I've worn one for years. When you're ready, I'd be happy to fit you for one."

I wondered what on earth could be involved in being *fitted* for one of these. Wasn't a woman an A, B, C or whatever? And did I even want one? Surely some women must choose to get on with their lives looking lopsided. But I didn't want to draw attention to myself. And I certainly didn't want to upset people.

I checked to make sure the foam prosthesis I'd selected had a price tag so that the young male cashier wouldn't be shouting around the store for a price check. Then I walked out of the pharmacy with a breast in a bag as if it were the most normal thing in the world.

"Let's have lunch," Katherine suggested.

"I don't know—it's already been quite a day."

"It would be good for you, a change of scene." She looked at me. "A nice meal at Chesa's?"

It seemed important to her. "Okay, let's go," I agreed.

When we arrived at Chesa's, the owner, Manuela, greeted us at the door. "And how are we today?" she asked, in her heavy European accent.

"Well, thank you, Manuela," I said. The restaurant was very busy. "Can you find room for us?"

"For you always—always find room." Manuela came up with a table in the middle of the restaurant and waved us to it. "Best

I can do," she shrugged. "Maybe a little noisy, but we have sweetbreads today. That will make up. Yeah?"

"It sure will."

I waited while Katherine decided what she wanted.

"Good, very good." Manuela nodded her head at me in a decisive fashion. "A Kahlúa and milk for you? Or maybe a nice glass of white wine?"

"Not today, thanks."

"You're working tonight," she said, as if she understood.

"No, not tonight."

"You're not well? I mean, you always have your Kahlúa and milk. When I see you coming I think, Oh, better I get out the Kahlúa and milk."

I laughed. "Just not drinking today. It happens, you know."

"Okay." She shrugged and walked away looking puzzled.

As always the food was excellent. I was enjoying it, but my eyes kept slipping over to a woman at the next table. I couldn't stop looking at her breasts. She wore a low-cut blouse that accentuated the heavy, ripe forms beneath. I was mesmerized.

In my whole life I had never wanted breasts like that. But now, suddenly, I did. For the first time I felt some understanding of how a woman who had lost a baby could think about stealing another woman's child. My feelings shifted back and forth between envy and loss.

"You look warm," Katherine said. "Maybe if you took off one or two layers of clothing—"

I put my fork down and asked Katherine if we could leave. The woman at the next table glared at me. I wanted to speak to her, offer some explanation, but I had no idea what I would say. "Sorry, but I love your breasts"? Or worse yet, "Would you mind if I held your breasts?"

I was in a cold sweat. I pushed myself away from the table. My head was full of the smell of coffee. The walls were moving as we worked our way between the tables.

Katherine pushed the door open, putting her hand under my elbow. "Are you all right?"

I didn't answer. My heart was pounding in my chest. The cool air made me feel the dampness on my skin. The traffic sounds mixed together into a strange hum. I grabbed for something to hold on to. Katherine pushed me down onto a bus-stop bench, and I leaned my head back.

"Put your head between your knees," she ordered.

I felt her hand gently rubbing my back. "Slow your breathing," she instructed. "That's better."

I concentrated on my breathing, then tried to slow my heart rate. I opened my eyes and looked at the ground. It stayed still. Slowly, I sat up and rested my head against a tree.

"I'm so tired," I said.

"You're not kidding," Katherine said. I could hear that she was worried.

"Good thing you're driving, eh?"

"Are you feeling any better?"

I nodded.

"Will you promise not to move while I get the car?"

I nodded again.

The next thing I knew, she was helping me into the car. I slept soundly all the way home.

11

WHEN I WOKE THE NEXT MORNING, the house was very quiet. There were times when I almost longed for the hospital. Now that I was home, no one called. Neighbours soundlessly came and went, leaving covered platters, casseroles and desserts at the door. I knew people were worried they might disturb me. They didn't want to intrude, and they knew my family would take wonderful care of me. But some dark side of me suspected I was a threat to them, too. I knew what must be going through their heads: if it can happen to you, it can happen to me. I figured there would be a lot of check-ups and mammograms going on in my circle of friends. And some of them must have felt relief that breast cancer had happened to me, not to them. I understood. I had experienced the same feelings as a paramedic.

I stayed in bed, feeling shooting pains in my nonexistent breast. Outside the bedroom window, a bank of black clouds had appeared over the mountains. The sky was threatening rain again. I picked up a book and read until the words on the page in front of me disappeared.

While I slept, a wind had come up, and the trees had turned dark and wet. Branches rubbed against the walls of the house. The forest moved.

Jenny, home from school, appeared in the doorway. When she saw I was awake, she slid under the quilt beside me.

"There's a card from Pat," Jenny said. "Why don't you call her?"

"I want to, but I guess I don't feel I have a lot to give right now."

"You're awesome, Mom—you always have a lot to give. You'd be totally pissed off with Pat if she used an excuse like that."

"So much wisdom from one so young," I said, tickling her until she bounced up and charged downstairs.

I went over and over what had happened in the restaurant. I haven't dealt with this, I admitted to myself. This goes much deeper than I imagined.

I wondered how long it would take to get back the strength I'd always been so proud of. I hated being unable to lift my arm more than a few inches from my body. There was nothing life-threatening about it, but there might as well have been for the anguish I felt. Putting on even a shirt or sweater wasn't easy. A pullover was impossible. And I was cold. Always cold.

I fantasized about marketing a new bra that had *DNR* embroidered on it. In the ambulance business, these initials stand for *Do Not Resuscitate*, or no heroic medical acts. I smiled to myself as I imagined the expression on a paramedic's face when my shirt was ripped open to start life-support. I even planned my funeral. Sunset. A baritone singing *Abide with Me* in an old candlelit church. "The darkness deepens," the hymn goes. And a party—oh, yes, a party.

My family and friends would be surprised I wanted a funeral. I wasn't religious, but I loved the cavernous emptiness of churches and was quite content to spend hours sitting in one. While I was in the hospital, many people had told me they were praying for my good health and even that whole con-gregations were in prayer. I took some comfort in other people's faith. But I wanted a funeral for another reason: I had not been allowed to attend my own father's service. I watched his burial from the shoulder of a nearby mountain. The ground was covered with snow. None of what I saw seemed remotely possible: the dark forms of family and neighbours hunched together as the winter's darkness descended upon his grave. I shouted my father's name, but no one heard.

I was almost asleep when Peter slipped into bed beside me. He pulled me close and kissed me. I drew away. Pain shifted soundlessly inside me. A few tears that had been lying in wait rolled down my cheek. Surgery, medications: I told myself that there were lots of obvious explanations for the way I felt. Eventually, I fell asleep.

I was wakened by my own movements. I felt very sore. It was still dark outside the window, although I had the sense that most of the night had passed. I felt around on the night table for my glasses and then went downstairs for a glass of water. The microwave clock read 04:30. I drank some water and swallowed two painkillers.

Light had started to appear in the sky. As I walked back upstairs, a bird began to sing.

When I woke again, everyone was gone. Peter had left a note saying that they'd decided to let me sleep. Katherine would be home at noon and Jenny would be working at the coffeehouse until late. Beside his note, there was a video he'd picked up from the university. It was Truffaut's *Jules and Jim*, which I needed to study for my course.

While I ate breakfast, I read the brochure about silicone prostheses that the woman at the pharmacy had given me. "This attachable breast form offers you more choices. Choice of shape, colour and size, but most important, choice of life-style.... You may begin your new world of freedom just as soon as you receive permission from your physician."

I sighed. "Enough of that already," I said to Freyja, who was lying by my feet. I invited her to watch the video with me.

Truffaut liked to depict a world that was devoid of logic, justice and order—just what I needed, I thought. His films maintained that it is the nature of love to be lost, but that to protect oneself from pain by not loving is not to live at all.

Jules and Jim was no exception. At first I was delighted by the triangle relationship between the woman and the two men, but it became more and more ominous as the film progressed. I knew I should not expect the happy ending so typical of American genre films, but when I watched the murder-suicide, the car plunging to its watery grave, tears streamed down my cheek. I sat alone in the stillness of the house, unable to stop crying. It wasn't the kind of crying that had me sobbing, but the tears kept coming. Perhaps it was simply a release. Perhaps it was some kind of delayed withdrawal from the morphine. I didn't know.

I heard tires on the gravel in our driveway. Katherine must be home. I didn't want her to see me like this, so I fled to the shower. I gasped as I looked down at where my breast should have been. Somehow I had managed not to really look at myself since the dressings had been removed. I looked at anything else I could: curtain, tiles, shower head. But this time, no matter what I looked at, I said over and over to myself: It's not there.

I washed myself the way I might have washed a stranger. I let the hot water pour over my right shoulder. Do something with yourself, I thought. I started to walk my fingers up the tile. I felt as though I were going to rip open. Gently, I touched the skin beneath the arm. It was hard to believe that an area where nerves had been destroyed could be so painful. The swelling made it look and feel sectioned like a quilt. The skin seemed thick, like rubber, and I felt the touch of my fingers on it the way you feel something through the sole of a shoe. I realized that a certain kind of familiarity with my body had been lost.

I'm normally a brave person, I reminded myself. I've canoed alone into the wilderness, climbed mountains and kayaked oceans. I've hauled people out of overturned trucks and burning cars. I've received a life-saving award for reacting under gunfire when a police officer was shot numerous times. Single-handedly, I've broken up street fights. I've had a dress torn to shreds when I tried to protect a woman who was being assaulted by another woman. While salvaging people's belongings after the slide that killed Pat's sons, I'd brought demolition to a halt by standing in front of a bulldozer. Although I had never thought of myself as fearless, it was a reputation I had earned.

So where was that person now, the one who kept smiling and looked on the bright side of things? Where was the woman who brought an attitude of adventure to everything she did? I missed her. I wanted her back. I stood forlornly in the shower and thought of her.

Still, the tears continued. I was helpless to stop them. I knew I had lost a great deal of blood, and I was weak. I knew that anaesthetics and drugs had mood-altering side effects. But there was something more happening to me, something I simply wasn't prepared for.

Wasn't it enough just to be alive? My breast was irrevocably and irretrievably lost, and I had to adjust to that fact. But the truth was, I felt cheated. I wanted to feel sexy again, and I was full of despair at the hopelessness of it. The scar was so ugly. If this surgery had been on my face, I wondered, would doctors have left such a horrendous scar?

Katherine stuck her head into the bathroom. "Are you okay?"

"Fine, thanks."

"You've been in the shower so long I thought I'd better make sure you hadn't drowned."

"I'll be out in a minute. The warm water just feels so nice."

"Call me if you want help."

The tears had not let up. Well, I thought, it looks as though I'm going to drown whether I'm in the shower or out of it. I took a long time to get dressed. I heard Katherine busy in the kitchen. When I finally went downstairs, I stood staring out the window. A hawk was wheeling over the trees.

"I picked up the library stuff you wanted," Katherine said. "Had to wander a labyrinth of stacks to find some of the books." I could feel her looking at me from the kitchen. I heard her put a bowl down on the counter and walk over to me.

"Mom, has something happened?"

Tearfully, I shook my head. She wrapped her arms around me, comforting me the way I had so often done for her as a child.

"Let the tears come," she said.

"I'm okay, you know. Honest. It's just that I can't find the tap to turn off the water."

"I love you, Mom."

I attempted a smile as I pulled away.

"I picked up the mail," she said softly. "There's another card from Pat. Are you going to call her pretty soon?"

She waited, giving me time to answer. I said nothing.

"How long have you been crying?" she asked.

"I'm *not* crying."

"Sorry, sorry—let me reword my question." And then we were both smiling.

"How long have you been ... like this?"

"Since I watched that video for my course."

"Oh, another *Hiroshima, Mon Amour*?"

"Actually, not nearly as devastating. Who knows ... a Mae West movie might have had the same effect on me today."

"Are you sleeping at night?"

"Not well—I keep dreaming."

"You're used to being so busy. You're used to being exhausted." She glanced at a book about cancer that I'd left on the table. "I think you need your crazy friends."

"One of these days, when I'm a little stronger, I'll call them."

"I'm not so sure you will."

I pulled off what I thought was a good-enough smile. "Pat calls Peter at work. He's told her I'm sleeping most of the time."

"And you ought to be resting more. I should never have suggested we have lunch."

"Listen, I feel like I'm doing nothing but sleeping. Anyway, lunch started out well. It's just that I kind of faded."

"That's for sure," she said, ruffling my hair.

She returned to the kitchen. Her back to me, she asked, "Has Deirdre called ... or dropped by?"

"No."

"I'd have thought she'd be around," she said quietly, as though talking to the cutting board.

I let out a long sigh. "She has things happening in her life too, you know."

Katherine didn't answer. She brought two salads to the table and sat down to eat lunch with me.

"Very salty lettuce," I said, flicking tears off the greenery.

She finished a mouthful and then looked at me. "You've been home a week—you need a plan."

"I have exercises to do, an exam to study for and research on breast cancer."

She rolled her eyes and continued to chew thoughtfully. "No, what I'm thinking of is something more physical. You need intensity. You only do well when things are challenging. Gruelling. Chaotic."

"This is challenging, sweetheart. Believe me, I see this as a challenge," I said. We laughed.

"To start with, come for a walk with Freyja and me after lunch."

"I can't go out like this. I'd leave a trail of tears behind me."

"Okay. Plan B. Get on the exercise bike and cycle a mile or two. Make yourself sweat. Get your endorphins going."

"Why do I have the feeling that things I've been saying to you over the years are being fed back to me?"

She grinned. "It's called revenge."

I considered her suggestion. Our exercise bike made you use your arms and legs for one of the best cardiovascular workouts possible. I referred to the bike as Leonardo, since it looked like something the artist might have designed. It had a huge fan for the front wheel, and the process of pushing the fan's long thin blades against air provided the workout.

I liked the idea in principle, yet I saw a problem. "I can't use my arms."

"So what you do is work twice as hard with your legs."

"I could give it a try."

"You'd better finish your tea first." Katherine grinned. "Or you might run out of fluid."

As Katherine cleared off the table, I gazed dreamily out the window. Now there was a pair of hawks circling low over the trees. Above them, a perfect and dazzling rainbow shimmered against a deep-blue sky.

I went upstairs for a rest. I lay on top of the quilt and said to myself: Nothing is happening to me that hasn't happened to thousands of other women.

I woke up confused, not knowing where I was for a moment. Someone was knocking on the front door. I waited for

Katherine to answer it, but the house remained silent. She must have taken Freyja for a walk.

I heard the door open, followed by Deirdre's shout. "Hey, anyone home?"

I grabbed some tissues to wipe away the tears but it seemed to be a lost cause. They were never-ending.

"I'm upstairs," I called out. "I'll be down in a minute." I put on my robe and walked downstairs in my bare feet.

Deirdre waited just inside the front door. When she saw me, she groaned. "Oh, you're dripping," she said, reaching out to give me a hug. "I thought you'd still be hiding behind that tan."

"I'm fine. Really. I'm not crying—I just can't stop the tears."

"Don't say you're fine to me. You're forgetting I'm from the 'fine' family too."

"Anyone can have a bad day." I smiled, holding my robe shut. "Actually, I feel quite happy."

"Being happy looks dangerous, my friend." She regarded me closely. "I think in this case it's kind of 'what you see is what you got.'"

"Not really." I shook my head. "Look, I can even smile."

"That's a smile, eh?"

I shrugged. "Do you want to come in? Have some tea? A drink?"

"I can't right now," she replied, sounding disappointed. "My family is in the car waiting. I just wanted to see how you were doing." She patted me gently on the cheek. "Not so well, I see."

I felt my left foot getting wet with tears. "Want to know something funny? I only have tears on my left side." I pointed at my right eye. "Look, it's dry."

"Trust you to be different," she said. She worked her tongue against her bottom lip. "Listen, I want you to know that I should have been around for you this past week—and I haven't been. I'm not going to make any excuses. I figure all I can do is say I'm sorry and try to do better in the future."

"It's not a problem, Deirdre." I felt the tears pour down my cheek.

She lifted her hand into the air and brushed my cheek dry with her sleeve. "That's what sleeves are for. Hasn't anyone told you that?"

I shook my head, smiling and trying to hold back tears at the same time.

"I have to go—everyone's waiting. But I'm going to call you tomorrow. Okay?"

I nodded, and we gave each other a hug. I closed the door behind her and then stood there, leaning against it. The car's engine had not been turned off, and I could hear it idling. I heard the sound of a car door slamming. The car started to back up. I caught myself wondering if I *would* hear from her tomorrow.

On the night table was Elaine's postcard. I stared through tears at the woman in the red armchair.

I had no idea how long I'd slept, but when I woke up, the bedroom was pitch-dark. I listened to rain pounding on the roof. I caught a whiff of Peter's pipe. At first, I thought it must be morning, and then slowly the house sounds told me it was evening. I got up and wrapped my robe tightly against my body.

Peter sat in his usual place at the dining room table. He held a *New Yorker* in his hands, but he was staring absently out the window. I slipped downstairs and put my arm around him in an affectionate headlock.

"Hello, Sleeping Beauty," he said, putting the magazine down. "I hear you've had a rough day."

"No, not really. My tear buckets are just too close to my eyes."

He stood up, and I walked into his arms, resting my head against his shoulder.

"Can I warm up some dinner for you?" he asked. "We ate a couple of hours ago."

"What time is it?" I asked, pulling away and looking at my watch. "My God, it's bedtime." I started to laugh.

"We made a family decision that you still need sleep more than food. I'll fix your dinner. Jenny wants you to go down to her room. She's studying."

"Where's Katherine?"

"Some of her university friends are in town—she's off somewhere with them."

Thinking of Katherine with her university friends was enough to make me let out a long sigh. I knew she had to be missing them. I walked down the stairs and paused outside Jenny's bedroom. I could smell incense. Quickly wiping the excess tears from my face, I knocked before opening her door. She waved to me. She was lying on her back on the bed, talking on the phone. She had one leg bent underneath the other and a shoe dangled from the foot of the leg on top. I waited while she said good-bye to her friend.

She jumped up and gave me a hug. "Hi, Mom, how are you?"

"Good, thanks," I answered. "How's it going?"

"Great, because it's spring and I'll soon be out of school—and because you're getting better. Aren't you?" she asked, warily eying my tears.

"I am indeed," I reassured her. "These tears are part of getting better."

She let her happy spirit take over again. After filling me in on what was happening with several of her friends, she told me she'd decided that eventually she wanted to go to art school.

"Once upon a time not so long ago you wanted to go to music school," I reminded her. "It's a long time since I've heard you practise the trumpet."

"I've cancelled my lesson for Saturday," she confessed. "I'm in a run to raise money for the Children's Fund. It won't hurt me to miss a lesson or two. My teacher says I play better than he does even when I don't practise."

"Don't count on that to last," I warned her lightly.

"You should see the silk painting I'm doing."

I knew she was trying to divert me, but I decided to let her get away with it.

"I'm so excited. It's taking me hours to colour in thousands of these tiny flowers, but it looks great."

"Why don't you bring it home and show me?" I suggested.

"Can't until it's finished—it's in a huge wooden frame so I've been working on it at lunch hour and after school."

Peter called to say dinner was ready. As I sat down at the table, I rooted around in my pocket for a tissue.

"Are you sure you're okay?" he asked.

"Yes. I just can't believe how weak I feel. I'm sorry I'm like this. I would never have thought it of myself."

"It's probably the blood loss on top of everything else." He smiled. "You may have to learn you're human." He kept me company while I poked at a trout that was trying to stare me down.

Dinner finished, I headed back to bed. The rain had stopped. I looked out the window. Amazingly, there was enough of a break in the clouds to see a full moon in a starless sky. I thought of the drowning scene at the end of *Jules and Jim*. I thought of a place a world away from here, where my mother and father had lived a life so painful that they had chosen to leave it. I tried to imagine what the last seconds of dying must feel like.

I almost drowned once when I was five or six years old. I didn't know how to swim. My family had a cabin at a lake. One hot day when we arrived at the lake, I watched my sisters run from the car straight into the water. I ran behind them, right over my head. I remember so clearly sitting on the bottom of the lake—just sitting there—until my father pulled me out and started to pump the water out of my lungs. The only part of the experience that was unpleasant was after I was hauled out of the water. Perhaps I hadn't realized that I was drowning as I drifted on the bottom of the lake, but afterwards I remembered with astonishing clarity that feeling of strange peacefulness. I didn't understand the violence of what my father was trying to do. I wanted him to stop. It was like a punishment. And I couldn't stop retching.

I remembered those moments on the bottom of the lake with almost a nostalgia. I'd always thought that if I ever needed to hasten my departure from the world, I knew how I would do it.

I fell asleep briefly, awakening to pain. I was soaked in sweat. I felt immersed in darkness. The house was silent. And then I heard Peter quietly breathing beside me. I had been dreaming again. I got up to remove the damp pyjamas. I slipped into my robe and went downstairs to my study. I turned on a small desk lamp and picked up a pen, releasing myself into endless dream darkness: *I woke in the dark, my heart pounding, knowing something had set me adrift ... the moon like a ship with lights ablaze ... going down into a sea heaving with blood and despair and rage, the waves hitting her broadside and flank, bearing her up just long enough for her cold indifferent spotlight to be held on the ghostly rowboats rocking in her wake ... and the women drowning, holding their children over their heads for rescue ... and I swimming right through them all.*

I put down the pen. The writing looked strange—cold and dark on the white sheet of paper. I touched the page with my fingers as if I might feel the words. Then I sat, gazing out the window. Moonlight reflected off the surface of the water. The sound of the distant ocean thundered inside my head.

12

WHEN I GOT UP IN THE MORNING, the ocean lay flat and still under a cloudless sky. Peter had already left for work. I remembered that Jenny had needed to be at school early to finish her art project. Katherine and Freyja were off on their morning walk. Although the tears had slowed down to a trickle, they were still there. I was feeling fragile enough to carry a box of tissues around the house and feared a shower might finish me.

By the time Katherine and Freyja got back, I'd managed to spend ten minutes on the exercise bike. According to the bike's computer, I'd travelled three miles.

"Way to go, Mom," Katherine said, pleased. "It even looks like you've got more sweat than tears."

"It might be a draw," I said, wiping my face with a towel. But it felt so good that I knew I was grinning.

"That worked so well, I'm going to try some sit-ups."

"Don't overdo it," Katherine warned, pulling Freyja away from my face as I got down onto the floor.

"I won't. I'm going to do a modified sit-up with my knees bent and my arms beside my body. Hold my feet down."

Katherine did as she was asked. "I don't know about this," she said.

"No problem," I said, heaving myself into a sitting position. I could feel the skin over my chest pulling. "Well, one is a start. Tomorrow, I'll try two."

The phone rang. Katherine reached for it and started talking while I stood up and dangled my arm around in small circles. I was amazed that I still had such limited mobility and range of motion.

Katherine held the telephone out. "It's Pat. Can you talk to her?"

I held the receiver in my left hand. "Hi," I said, proud that my voice sounded full of energy.

"Rosalind, my friend," I heard her say, her voice musical and hearty. "I was just phoning to see how you were doing. Katherine said you are in the middle of exercises. You never cease to amaze me. Do you want to call me back?"

"No, I'm finished. Thanks for the cards, Pat."

"Well, you know something? Everyone has been calling me for reports on you. I've been phoning Peter at work and he said you sleep an awful lot, so none of us wanted to disturb you. But I decided to call anyway. Rosalind, I have a little favour to ask of you."

"Oh, oh," I said, recognizing her tone of voice.

"We want to party. And we want to party with you. Now I realize this may not exactly be what the doctor has prescribed. But as you know, you have responsibilities to your friends. We all miss you. So here's the plan. We come to you. We bring everything. You don't have to do a thing but put up with us for a short while."

There was a long silence on the line.

"Boy, you've sure knocked me over with your enthusiasm," she said, laughing.

"I don't know, Pat. I'm still feeling a bit like a blob."

"The word is blimp, my sweet. Much more elevating." She added in a serious voice, "Roz, you're not feeling *down*, are you?"

Her question took me back to a difficult period after the slide when I had asked her if she was depressed. She had answered, "Rosalind, we don't say 'depressed' in our family. It's too negative. People are allowed to feel down. Not depressed."

"Just a touch," I said now, and then tried to explain it away. "I feel so terribly weak—"

"Roz, you can't get *depressed* on us. We need you."

I laughed. She always had a wonderful way of twisting everything just slightly.

"Can I do anything?"

"No, I'm coming along. Really I am."

"Listen, maybe a visit from us *is* what you need. We won't stay long. I promise."

"When were you thinking of?"

"Tomorrow? Around lunchtime?"

Knowing how much I'd missed the chatter and craziness, I said, "That would be great."

"Wonderful," she answered. "I'm bringing your favourite soup."

"The one with all the scallops and shrimp? The one that is so expensive you have to take out a second mortgage just to buy the ingredients?"

"The very same," she said.

"I can't wait. Who's coming?"

"It won't be a cast of thousands. Half a dozen of us? Can you handle that?"

I laughed. "A half-dozen of you guys is like a hundred of any other group."

"In the meantime, I'm sending some little angels down Howe Sound to be with you."

"I'm looking out the window, Pat." I watched light play across the ocean. "I see them."

"Good. I've instructed these celestial cheerleaders to stay with you for a while. Till tomorrow, then. Bye."

Smiling, looking for angels, I stood at the window watching the sun pour down light. A prawn boat was cutting slowly across the water, setting out its traps in a string.

"Katherine, I'm going to lie down. Please don't feel you have to be quiet. I can sleep with just about anything going on."

"I was thinking of going out. Allison is in town," she explained. "If you don't think you need me for anything?"

"Not a thing. Go and have a good time. I'll be fine."

When I woke up, the house was still quiet. I could sense I was alone except for Freyja, who was luxuriating in the sunlight coming through the window.

I was heartened to notice that my face was dry. I got up and made myself some tea, then nibbled at a tabouli salad Katherine had left for me.

The sun called me, mug in hand, onto the deck outside. I took a deep breath, smelled the air and touched some daring crocuses. Despite the cool air, I felt the sun's warmth on my skin. I wrapped myself in a blanket and dozed for some time in a lawn chair. When the sun left the deck, I went back inside to sit at my desk and think over my day.

What I had accomplished with my exercises and the telephone conversation wasn't much, but it was enough to encourage me to keep moving and to take one day at a time. It seemed important to keep inhaling the thick, wonderful scent of flowers, becoming heady on the nothing that a breath is.

Deirdre hadn't called. Normally it wouldn't matter. I'd

know that she was busy. But when I could do little but sit around and look out windows, suddenly it did matter. "My problem—not hers," I said to the ocean.

I understood that it took time to adjust to a diagnosis like cancer. But I was torn between a desire to just get on with my life and a need to understand the disease. I had no desire to see myself as a victim, and that was the way much of what I read made me feel. I wanted only to grow stronger and put the experience behind me. Yet I needed to know and understand the enemy. And once I knew the enemy, I needed to know how to fight back. Finding out about the breast cancer had led me to know my own mortality in a way I never had before. Cancer might have killed me. It might still—unless I learned how to live with it.

In my research so far, I had come up with more questions than answers. Countless times I had read that breast cancer is considered the most unpredictable of all cancers. There are known causes for many other types of cancer, but not this disease. The best anyone seemed to have come up with was that either an inherited factor or a carcinogen creates a mutation in a normal gene, then something else comes along and causes a second mutation. When this second mutation occurs, you possess the gene for cancer. But it was all guesswork.

I pulled out some of the medical journals and magazines Katherine had picked up for me. I wrote a few notes on a piece of paper. The more I read, the more it seemed as though some of the answers might lie in factors we knew nothing about. I felt cold. I decided I had done enough for one afternoon. I put my pen down and went upstairs for a rest.

Freyja was on the bed beside me when I woke. Since I had been home she was taking every opportunity to stay away from her bed by staying on ours. I put my hand out to rub her gently behind the ears. She looked back at me and stretched, nearly sending me onto the floor.

"Okay, okay," I told her. "I'm getting up."

Excited by the prospect of dinner, Freyja tagged along behind me. I fed her and then decided it was time for my arm exercises. I liked to do whatever I could to delay them, because they hurt. I decided to have a shower; the exercises went better if I did them with a torrent of hot water on my shoulder and arm. I dangled my arm and moved it around in little circles, then walked my fingers up the small square tiles. Hmm, I thought, maybe one tile higher today? I felt better. I was not quite singing in the shower yet. Still ...

When I got out, I gently patted the sore parts of my body dry with a towel. I could smell onions cooking. And garlic. I went downstairs to find Peter preparing dinner. He had an apron on, and as usual he looked totally at home in the kitchen.

"How was your day?" I asked.

"Too busy, but otherwise fine. How about yours?"

"Better," I said. "I'm doing better."

"Good," he answered warmly, fussing with a sauce. "Anything happen around here today?"

"Pat called. She and a few of the girls are coming over at lunchtime tomorrow."

"Do you feel you're ready for that?"

"I think so. I miss everyone. Pat said they were bringing everything. Hey, I even spent some time on the bike today and did a sit-up."

"Don't overdo it," he cautioned.

"One sit-up?"

He smiled and put dinner on the table. "Would you like some wine?" he asked, holding the bottle above a glass.

"No, thanks—not just yet."

"Where is everyone?" I asked, realizing that this was another role reversal. Normally, I was the one who knew where Katherine and Jenny were.

"Both of them left messages on the answering machine. I guess you were in the shower. They're going to be late."

As I cleaned my plate, I realized that I hardly ever knew where Jenny was these days. I didn't expect Katherine to report in, but even when I was working, I expected Jenny to keep in touch by calling me on my pager.

I watched the erratic flight of a few bats as they zipped back and forth in front of the dining room window. I thought of the bat house that Peter hadn't had time to build.

"Did Jenny say where she was?" I asked.

"At Tegan's."

"Oh, good," I said, relieved. Her friend lived just down the road.

"Actually, I called too, wondering if you wanted me to pick anything up."

I nodded. "We are probably going to have to replace our hot water system. My showers are getting longer and longer, but they feel so good."

After dinner, Peter took Freyja out for her evening walk. I picked up another article from my stack and started to read: "People assume that the cancer cell is an aggressive and powerful intruder capable of ravaging the body. Cellular biology tells us the opposite. A cancerous cell is a weak and confused cell. The immune system is composed of many specialized cells which are designed to attack and destroy all weak and confused cells in the body on an ongoing basis. This includes tumour cells. For cancer to occur, the immune system must be inhibited in some way. Many researchers now believe that childhood loss, and the effects of emotional stress—particularly chronic stress—can suppress the immune system, thus disarming the body's natural defences against cancer. The enemy cells are not destroyed by the army of white blood cells, and so these enemy cells claim some part of the body for themselves."

I tossed the magazine aside. I walked upstairs and pulled the covers up to my chin, trying to stop my brain from going over and over everything I had read.

When Peter came to bed he pulled me close. His hands drifted over my body, touching all the right places. I pulled away. Without a word he turned towards the other side of the bed.

I lay awake, staring out the window. The moon rose in the night like a flawless pearl.

Trying to avoid the restless tossing and turning was a futile effort. I slipped quietly out of bed, picking up my robe and slippers. In the study, I turned on my desk lamp. I stared for a long time at the blank sheet of paper.

As I ate breakfast the next morning, I made anagrams out of the words on the back of the cereal box. By the time Katherine came back from walking Freyja, I had folded laundry, done the dishes and ironed a shirt or two.

"Don't start cleaning the house," she warned me. "I have everything organized."

"Not to worry. It's about time I do something useful around here."

She took the iron out of my hand. "Don't start ironing, either. Knowing how you feel about that job I'll start to worry that you've completely cracked."

I carried my coffee out onto the deck and tried to get a feel for the kind of day it was going to be. I was nervous about people coming for lunch. I'd been out of service, and I worried that I wouldn't be up to performing the way I'd expect of myself. I looked at the sky and wished that the sun would shine.

I went upstairs and selected a silk shirt. I turned sideways in the mirror to see how it hung. It looked fine. Katherine came upstairs, her arms loaded with clothing that had been left here and there in the house.

"You look absolutely beautiful," she said, as she dropped her armful on the bed.

I smiled appreciatively at her, then headed off to bring some wine up from the basement. I managed to carry three bottles in one trip. Two went into the refrigerator, and I poured myself a drink from the third.

"Does the house pass?" Katherine asked, pausing in mid-flight on the stairs.

"It does. Thanks, Katherine."

"Okay, I'm gone," she said. "I'm going to look for a job while your friends are here."

"Then you've definitely decided against returning to university?"

"Don't belabour it, Mom," she warned gently. "Remember, no one—" and I joined in so that we said it together "—can teach you about life."

It was shortly before noon when Pat burst through the door carrying baskets overflowing with food, flowers and wine.

"Hello, my sweet," she said magnanimously, putting everything down so that we could give each other a hug. She stood back and looked at me. "You're looking very trim," she winked, and we both laughed at the pun.

She began to sing the lyrics of "We're Here for a Good Time ... Not a Long Time" but was interrupted as the rest of the gang pushed their way in, talking and laughing, each in turn waiting impatiently to give and receive attention.

Marilyn arrived at the bottom of the steps, screaming, "Rozzie, do something with your monster dog." Someone had let Freyja out, and she was doing a jumping thing she was fond of. When I got to Freyja, she was smiling, showing her teeth. Marilyn was backed against the railing, trying to reason with her. "Good doggie, nice doggie. Do you talk? Couldn't we discuss this?"

Back inside, Donna pulled a tablecloth out of a basket and set the table; Sylvia put a casserole dish in the oven; Marcia opened bottles of Far Niente wine from her own vineyard in the Napa Valley. Roberta was in the kitchen, complaining that her dessert wasn't co-operating, and Deirdre stood beside her, throwing a Caesar salad together. I had to shout to be heard over the noise. "You guys bring a whole new dimension to Meals on Wheels."

Pat was so purposefully busy and energetic in the kitchen that I half-expected her to knock something over. She stirred a huge pot of soup and left it to simmer on the stove. Next, she placed a baked salmon on the table. The wine and baguettes sticking out of one basket made me think of a porcupine. In the middle of the table, there was a block of ice with roses frozen inside it. Pat handed me serviettes with small pictures of Leonardo's Mona Lisa. In the first frame, the Mona Lisa's facial expression was the same as in the original masterpiece, but as my eyes moved along frame by frame, the famous woman gradually broke out into a great grin.

Pat momentarily stopped her bustling to bring over a basket. From beneath a tea towel, like a magician's dove, she pulled out a bottle of Kahlúa. "May I pour you a Brown Cow?"

"Actually, I have a glass of wine."

She startled everyone with the volume of her, "What?"

"Not to worry, after this glass I'll be into the Kahlúa. Count on me."

"I'm so relieved," she said, giving me a pat on the head. "I worried for a minute that you had changed on us." I tried to follow her into the kitchen, but she put her hand up like a police officer stopping traffic and ordered me to sit down.

The sun suddenly broke through the clouds, and the light-starved group unanimously agreed that the luncheon should move outside. Everyone talked at once, picking up dishes of food and bottles of wine, heading out onto the large deck.

I savoured every mouthful of Pat's soup and went back for a second helping. Donna, Sylvia and I—three women who had experienced cancer—sat at one end of the table. Pat must have read my thoughts, because I suddenly heard her say, "Oh, oh, that's the bad end of the table—just look who's sitting there." I laughed at Deirdre, who squirmed dramatically towards Pat.

"Isn't it amazing," Pat said. "Three of us here today have had to deal with cancer." There was an air of seriousness for just a moment until she jumped up. "Where's my camera? I'd better get a picture in case someone doesn't make it to the next luncheon."

"You know something," I said, looking from one face to the next, "I just realized that the seven of us have a total of twenty-one daughters."

"Marcia having six kind of tips the scale," Marilyn said.

Pat interrupted everyone's laughter by stepping back outside with her camera waving in the air. "Closer together, everyone," she instructed. "Sickos with the healthy ones—that's better." I heard the shutter click. I imagined the photograph, seen already as if in a frame, and I wondered who was next.

When Pat put her camera down, she raised her wine glass in a toast. "To good friends, and to our good health." She placed her hand over her mouth. "Whoops, sorry," she laughed, patting me on the head again.

I smiled when I heard Marcia say to Marilyn, "I can't believe what comes out of that woman's mouth."

Marilyn waved her fork wildly in the air. "It's Rozzie's own fault. Rozzie wanted us to keep a sense of humour. And you know Pat." Marilyn rolled her eyes. "Nothing in moderation."

Donna laughed. "You've got to admit, she does have style."

I looked around at my friends and thought how wonderful it was to be with them again. I had missed the silliness and hilarity.

Deirdre came up behind me, gave my shoulders a gentle squeeze and said, "Come and talk."

I followed her to a two-seater. She patted the cushion beside her. She wore a low-cut black blouse, and I realized that even my friends were fair game for my breast envy.

"So," she said, "and don't tell me fine, how are you doing?"

"On a scale of one to ten—all things being relative—I'd place myself at about an eight. Not too bad, I'd say."

"Not bad at all," she agreed, studying her drink. For a moment, she seemed slightly vague, abstracted—lost in her private thoughts. Then she said, as if to herself, "You're amazing. I don't know how you've survived what you've gone through."

"You just do," I said, smiling back at her.

It felt good to be sitting beside her again, talking. I wanted to say: Deirdre, I've missed you. Her name had sounded so loudly in my mind that I wondered if I had spoken it, but she showed no reaction. I said, "What's happening in your life?"

"Nothing much," she said. "The usual rushing about."

My fingers pulled idly at a few weeds in a planter. "You still feeling tired?"

"Me?"

"Yes."

"I'm fine," she said with surprising intensity.

I could not decipher her look, but I knew instinctively that the conversation was over, its loose ends left to hang. Everything seemed fragile and held together by silence. But into that empty space rushed voices, the clinking of ice, someone breaking up with laughter. Marilyn was impersonating an old boyfriend. I couldn't hear exactly what she was saying but I laughed too when I saw her clasp her neck with both hands as if she'd been garroted. Deirdre and I talked about inconsequential things until the sun went behind a tree, leaving us in the shade. I shivered.

"Cold?" she asked, picking up Pat's sweater and wrapping it around my shoulders. "Let's move back into the sun," she suggested, dragging our chair into the centre of the group. "Here," she said. "Why don't you stretch out?"

The warmth felt good on my right side. Everyone was talking at once. I felt the sun cover me like a blanket.

I gave a start. Everything was silent. I heard a page turn.

Pat sat quietly in a chair, glancing through a magazine.

"Where is everyone?" I asked incredulously, pushing a blanket back.

"Home, my dear. You fell asleep."

"I'm so sorry."

"Don't be," she said, waving away my apology. "I'm just sorry you didn't get to see everyone tiptoeing out of here. It was hysterically funny. I think they made more noise than when they arrived, but it didn't wake you. I've been having a wonderful time sitting here in the sun reading."

I looked around the deck. "Amazing. They even cleaned up before they left. I didn't hear a thing."

"Well, on your birthday we set a record for the longest luncheon ever." She winked at me. "It's fitting that today we record the shortest one."

I stretched and stood up.

"Hi, Mom," Katherine called from the dining room.

"Hi, darling. How long have you been home?"

"I arrived just as the herd of giggling women stampeded."

"Did you find a job?"

"Yes," she said, sounding forlorn.

"It's that bad, is it?" Pat asked.

"Waitressing."

"Big bucks, Katherine," Pat said, trying to cheer her up.

"That's the only reason I'm doing it."

Pat stood up and gave me a hug. "I'm out of here, beauty. Katherine is giving me a ride. I'll call tomorrow."

I stayed outside, quietly thinking over the day, watching Freyja vacuum up bits of food left over from lunch. I reviewed everything Deirdre and I had said to each other. She had been warm and caring. Perhaps I was imagining her inaccessibility.

13

I WOKE TO FIND Katherine putting a handful of wildflowers into a vase beside my bed. She looked down at me with her sky-blue eyes. "Sorry to wake you, Mom, but your doctor's appointment is in an hour."

Sunlight streamed in through the window. I stared at my watch in disbelief—fourteen hours of sleep. Peter had come home and gone back to work without my knowing. In the short time it took me to get ready, the sky was threatening rain again.

My appointment was with Duncan. I tried to think of questions I should ask.

Sitting in the waiting room, I watched a woman breastfeed her baby. She looked up and saw me watching. I smiled, and she smiled back.

I didn't have to wait long until the nurse called my name. "Hi, Rosalind," she said, warmly grasping my hand. "I hear you've been a model patient."

I smiled, feeling pleased.

"Will Duncan be examining you today?" she asked.

"No, I don't think so. He asked me to come in for a talk."

"I'll put you in his office, then."

Duncan came in right away with a cheerful, "Hi, how are you today?"

"On the mend," I said.

"Good for you. How's the pain?"

"It's there, but it's manageable. There's this tight feeling all the time."

He opened my chart. "That feeling will be there for several months while the healing takes place—like the pain, it will gradually subside."

"What about the numbness?"

"Nerves regenerate very slowly. Give it time. I'd say that whatever numbness you have after six to eight months is probably about what you'll be left with."

"And the phantom pains?"

He smiled. "Some women report phantom pains years afterwards."

"But that's good," I said.

He looked questioningly at me.

"That means those women are still alive."

He nodded. "Let's see how the incision looks."

"I guess I'm lucky I'm not a large-breasted woman."

"It's all relative," he answered, catching my eye. "It's not any easier for you than for any other woman." I undid the buttons of my shirt. Without touching me, he studied my incision. Then he walked back to his desk. "That's quite a scar you're getting—part of the tightening you feel is scar tissue adhering to your chest wall."

"I've been rubbing aloe vera and Vitamin E on the incision."

"Good. Soon we'll start you on some physiotherapy—laser treatment will help soften up that tissue."

"Can we talk statistics for a moment?"

"What are you wondering?"

"Can you throw any numbers on what my chances of survival are now that I've had the surgery?"

He looked at me for a moment without saying anything. "Frankly, I'd rather not. Survival times are statistical terms of probability—nothing more. Anyone who is diagnosed with cancer, their first question is, 'How long have I got?'"

I nodded.

"What I am suggesting is that you ignore the statistics and just make up your mind that you are going to be a survivor."

"On an intellectual level, I'm in complete agreement. However, those percentages for recurrence roll around in the back of my mind—"

"Get them out of your mind," he interrupted. "For a few years, every ache and pain you have will make you fear that it's cancer. That's a normal reaction—it will take two to five years before you regain some faith in your body."

"What if there are pains in the bones? I'm a little paranoid about cancer spreading to my bones. It can have my liver and my brain," I attempted to joke.

He smiled. "Being a little paranoid is probably like being a little pregnant. Have you got pains in your bones?"

I shook my head. "No."

"You've just had the bone scan, which was negative."

"Yes, but I understand that a bone scan only shows a tumour if the cancer is quite advanced."

"That's true. But if it gives you peace of mind, we can take another scan a few months from now and compare." He paused and wrote some notes in my file.

"If a pain develops in one of my bones, is there a way of knowing whether or not it might be cancer?"

"There are no hard and fast rules. As a guideline, I'd say that if a pain is constant, the possibility of metastasis is there. If the pain comes and goes, it's probably not cancer." He put his pen down. "I know it's easier said than done, but what I tell any woman who has had breast cancer is to try to keep a watchful eye on herself without becoming obsessed."

He leaned back in his chair. "From everything I've observed, you have been incredibly strong throughout all of this. I also know what this kind of a diagnosis does to people. Am I reading you correctly, or are you having some difficulties?"

I teared up a little as I answered. "I think I'm doing well and yet ... I mean, this is not how I'm used to seeing myself. I can't believe how weak I am. I'm not flat-on-my-back weak, but I want to sleep all the time." I managed a smile. "I had to sit all of two minutes in your waiting room and I was already looking at the floor thinking how nice it'd be to conk out right on the spot. Maybe I have narcolepsy."

"You should be doing nothing but resting right now. I wish rest cost money, because then I could prescribe it and people would believe in it."

A few tears rolled down my cheek. I pointed to them. "Look—no tears on the right side of my face."

He leaned forward to see for himself.

"Interesting, wouldn't you say?"

"Very. Women often don't perspire under their arms on the same side as a node excision, but this is definitely interesting."

"You know, it's strange. I've never actually cried throughout this whole ordeal, but for the last few days I've teared up enough to upset my electrolyte balance."

"Well, you've been very stoic. Some women cry, shout or scream in this office when they receive the news you've received. Remember that there's a place for yelling and screaming. Sometimes it can actually help."

I smiled, deciding to move onto safer ground. "How long do you think it will be until I can drive?"

"As long as it takes to get your arm working again. Maybe a month?"

I closed my eyes. "You know, I can't help but feel that part of my problem is that there seems so little I can do to help myself. I rode on my exercise bike yesterday. I also did a single sit-up with my hands down beside my body. I can't rip apart, can I?"

"You should be fine. Just don't get carried away and throw your hands behind your back."

"No chance of that," I said, showing him the small arc my arm could swing through without pain.

"Let your body tell you what you can do. If something hurts, don't do it." He glanced at me but seemed hesitant to speak. Then he said, "There is a group of women who get together once a month in this area. They have all had breast cancer. It's a support group. I highly recommend you go to their meetings."

I shook my head. "No, I'm not ready for that. I'm not ready

to belong to a group where the common denominator is cancer. I'd need to be stronger before I could do that."

We were both silent for a moment. I studied my hands. There was the sound of rain hitting the windows. When I looked up, he gave me a gentle smile. "It's not hard for all this rain to dampen spirits, you know."

"One day it's spring, and the next day it's winter," I replied, starting to put on my jacket.

He stood up and helped me slip it on. He stepped back and reached for the door handle, but he didn't open the door. "You have come through all of this exceptionally well. You know that, don't you?"

"So I keep being told." I looked directly at him. "What I'd like to know is, what do women do who live in rural areas and don't have a choice of hospitals and top-notch doctors? What do they do without bookstores and libraries and support groups? What do they do if they don't have good friends and caring families?"

I looked at his hand on the door handle. "There's something else that bothers me," I said. "Some researchers seem to be pointing the finger at screwed-up childhoods, emotional losses and stress as causes of breast cancer. How much of a connection do you think there is?"

He leaned against the door. "I've always thought theories that diseases are caused by a mental state and can be cured by a mental state are an indication of how much is not understood about that particular disease." He folded his arms in front of him. "However, I certainly believe stress can inhibit the immune system, which can make a person more susceptible to disease. Stress is part of everyone's life, but it's been observed that an awful lot of women who have breast cancer are under chronic stress and have disturbances in their home and work lives."

"What about the connection with loss?"

"Breast cancer in general is connected with loss—loss of a breast, loss of something that is one of the ways our society defines femininity, loss of a way of life, loss of a sense of security." He paused. "What I would suggest is that you set yourself up in what you think is an ideal environment for healing. Identify what causes stress to you and try to minimize it."

He looked at me questioningly, and I nodded.

When he opened the door, I headed out through a waiting room packed with people. I knew my appointment had been for a half-hour visit, and I suspected my doctor had been generous with me at a cost to some of these people. I saw Katherine leaning against the wall. Her arms were folded and she was gazing out the door, daydreaming.

"Ready?" she asked, startled, when she realized I was standing beside her.

The rain was coming down hard, and I actually ran for the car. As we drove along the rain-splashed streets, I eyed a toy store and asked Katherine to stop.

"Something I can pick up for you?"

"If you don't mind." I handed her my wallet. "I'd like a nerf ball—about this big," I said, making a grapefruit-sized circle with my hands.

She returned in no time. "Mission accomplished," she said, throwing me the ball. "I chose yellow—the colour of the sun."

"Perfect," I said, starting to squeeze the ball with the fingers of my right hand.

Katherine glanced at me every time we stopped at a red light. "Is that hard to do?" she asked seriously.

"It just takes a little concentration. I can feel it right up my arm."

"Well, don't overdo it," she cautioned, and we laughed.

When we got home, the green light was blinking on the answering machine. I pushed the playback button. "Good morning, good morning. And how are we this morning?" Pat's voice called out. "I had such a good time yesterday. Hope you're not paying for it today. Give me a call. Bye." The machine beeped and then I heard Deirdre's voice. "Good morning—thought I'd just call to see how you're doing. Talk to you soon. Bye." Beep. Peter's voice came on next, letting me know that he had to work over the weekend. I heard, "Love you," and the machine clicked off.

"I'm off to work," Katherine said. "You need anything?"

"No thanks, sweetheart."

I phoned Pat and Deirdre, ate some leftovers from the party and settled at my desk to write a poem. I placed the sheets of paper in front of me, staring at their taunting blankness for a long time.

Freyja, finding a sunny niche in the corner of the room, decided to join me. I gave up on trying to write and decided that I might as well dig into some more of my research on the causes of breast cancer. The hours ticked past. Although I felt tired, I was reassured to find I could stay with it.

Recently, the spotlight had been on high-fat foods as the most probable cause of breast cancer. Yet no one was sure whether the danger was from all fats, animal fats alone, or the fat from animals treated with hormones or given feed treated with pesticides. I made a mental note to take a serious look at my diet. I loved to steal fat trimmings off other people's plates. I loved chicken skin and beef rind. And butter. And cheese. Then there was my favourite drink, Kahlúa and milk. I couldn't help smiling when I thought of all the teasing I'd had over the years about my healthy drink. There seemed to be little argument that breast cancer rates were highest in prosperous countries where people ate refined and processed foods high in fats, additives and sugar. Yet surely, I thought, diet can hardly be the only answer: the majority of fat-eating North Americans did not have breast cancer.

Another study pointed the finger at alcohol consumption, arguing that if you had more than three drinks a week, you were more likely to develop breast cancer. I stopped reading, glancing at Freyja on the floor. She had nudged me with her paw, giving me a sudden sorrowful look.

A third study found that pesticide levels were higher in the fat tissue of women who had breast cancer than in the tissue of those who did not. I shifted uneasily in my chair. I had spent my childhood in the Okanagan Valley at a time when DDT was revered as a wonder chemical. We used to play under fruit trees that were dripping with it. This same paper mentioned that breast cancer in Israel dropped 30 per cent following an aggressive program to phase out organochlorine pesticides.

Almost all researchers agreed that hormonal levels of estrogen played an important role in the development of breast cancer. Women who had never been pregnant seemed to be more at risk. It appeared that the more children you'd had—and the earlier the better—the less at risk you were. Researchers theorized that the more menstrual periods a woman had over a lifetime, the more prone she was to breast cancer. I had been twenty-four when I had the first of my two children, but I had no idea how old I'd been when I had my first period. One recent study boasted that there were virtually no cases of breast cancer in women who'd had complete hysterectomies at a young age. Twelve years earlier, I had undergone a hysterectomy to remove a troublesome uterus. The surgeon did not remove my ovaries. That had seemed like a good decision then, but now I wondered what it might have cost me.

I settled more deeply into my chair. Since our own hormones affected our risk of developing breast cancer, it stood to reason that hormones such as estrogen in birth control pills might also have an effect. There was certainly a correlation between the time the pill had been around and the increase in the incidence of breast cancer. I should have known *that* would come home to roost—I had taken the pill for years. But I read that the pill had changed so much in its components over the years that studies about a possible causal relationship tended to contradict each other.

As I turned pages, Freyja eyed me intermittently. At one point I dropped my pen, and she studied it closely. Eventually she closed her eyes, lost to the chases and smells of her dreams.

I continued with my reading. Another study reported that women who had experienced acute postpartum mastitis— inflammation of the breast while nursing—had an increased risk of breast cancer. I started a personal list of risks and put a check-mark beside that one too. It didn't surprise me when I read that 80 per cent of women who get breast cancer weren't considered high-risk before the diagnosis.

That there was a link between radiation and an increased risk of breast cancer seemed to be agreed upon by almost everyone in the field. The risk was believed to go up in proportion to the amount of exposure. I remembered the fluoroscopes that were so popular when I was a child. You could slip your feet into this eerie green space and see the outline not only of the new shoes you were trying on but also of your bones. Whenever someone in my family went to town, I would tag along just so I could see the bones of my feet move in the big magical box. I thought of all the times my teeth had been X-rayed and the accumulated radiation from other X-rays over the years.

I read that breast cancer rates are 6.5 times higher in countries with nuclear waste sites. Researchers who had studied breast cancer in the survivors of the atomic explosions in Hiroshima and Nagasaki found the increase of the disease to be far more dramatic among women who were in their teens and early twenties at the time of the bombing. This fit the theory that the developing breast is particularly vulnerable to carcinogenic agents, perhaps because of greater hormonal activity in the body. There was something else that was interesting here, too. These studies also identified breast cancer's long latency period; despite exposure, the disease did not normally appear until a woman was approaching middle age. I remembered the line from *Hiroshima, Mon Amour*: "What we know of as part of our past will be part of our future."

When Jimmy Carter was president of the United States, more than a thousand people were awarded damages from the government for cancers caused by the nuclear testing in Nevada. The award was reversed by a higher court, which decided that the government was not responsible for what had happened. The previous year I had read a book called *Refuge* by American writer Terry Tempest Williams. How many had she said it was? Seven of nine women in her family with breast cancer—and no cancer history before all those above-ground atomic tests in Nevada, where she lived as a child. It really gave new meaning to the expression "depending on which way the wind blows." I remembered reading that the fallout from those tests left animals dead in their tracks. Since then, there had been Three Mile Island and Chernobyl.

I looked around the house. From my study I could see a microwave, a television, a smoke alarm, an illuminated clock, insulation in an unfinished wall, chemically treated wood, a diet cola, appliances run by electricity, my computer. I had

always thought of our home in the forest as being inviolable—
a place of sanctity. Maybe it was the most dangerous place in
the world.

Freyja jumped up as Peter opened the door to the study.
Patting her on the head, he looked at me. "It's good to see you
working at your desk."

"It's felt good to be doing it."

"How are the sniffles today?" he asked. "You seem to be
doing much better."

"I am," I agreed, just a little frightened that to say I was
stronger might invite sudden collapse.

Peter and I discussed what I had been reading while he took
off his jacket and shoes. I noticed that he had two different-
coloured socks on. I made a mental note to do some laundry.

When he wandered into the kitchen, I settled back into my
own silence, considering how much I had learned since my
breast cancer had been diagnosed. I had been exposed to just
about every risk that threatened a breast cancer patient, and
previously I had considered myself the least likely candidate
for such a disease. The statistics—and everything I read—were
telling me that it was probably a combination of risks and
exposures that brought about the current epidemic. All indica-
tions were that this was a disease associated with the toxic
effluvia of an industrial economy that created affluence, a
disease associated with excess. Even if a cure were discovered,
major changes in the way we lived our lives would be necessary
to end the ravages of breast cancer.

The more research I did, the more I believed that no one
won with this disease. There were a few variables: how quickly
the diagnosis was made; how aggressive the breast cancer was,
and its location in the breast; some decisions regarding treatment. Early diagnosis sometimes bought time in a big way, but

not always. The best I could come up with was a feeling that if I survived five years, my chances of living long enough for something else to kill me became better and better.

I heard Peter working his whisk briskly in a large copper bowl. I walked over to him. "You're making a soufflé?"

"Trying—it's gotten a little out of control. Could you stir the egg yolks with the pureé?"

"What's in the pureé?" I asked, gently stirring.

"Leftovers."

I watched as he folded my mixture into his glistening whites—lifting the batter up, over and under, without losing the air he'd so carefully beaten into them.

14

IT WAS SATURDAY MORNING. I was aware of quiet activity downstairs but continued to doze until the house was still. I felt very sore and wondered if I had rolled onto my side in my sleep. As I lay there, I took a family inventory. Peter had probably already gone to work for the day. Katherine was working too. And Jenny? Why had she slept at her friend Jen's place last night? I couldn't remember. I brooded briefly on my post-surgical memory.

I made my way downstairs. Standing in the dining room, I swallowed two pills and read a note left on the table. "Dear Mom, please do not feed Freyja. No matter what she tells you, she has been fed. Love you, Katherine." Underneath, Peter had sketched a drawing of the dog begging for food.

Freyja cocked her head. She looked over to where her food was stored, then back at me. "Forget it," I said, giving her a hug.

While I ate breakfast, I held the nerf ball and squeezed it from time to time. I washed the dishes by hand before wiping the table with slow circular movements. Chores done, I walked down to the piano and sat on the stool. The keys were at a perfect height for my right hand. Although my fingers were already fatigued from squeezing the nerf ball, I played a quiet Bach piece, moved into Schumann's *Träumerei*, and then crashed and burned while attempting Tchaikovsky's demanding *None but the Lonely Heart*. I couldn't play another note, but I had a smug feeling of accomplishment.

The indifferent sun, shining one minute and disappearing the next, threw sudden light onto the house. I sat on the exercise bike but felt too sore to do much. Listening to Satie's *Gymnopédie* seemed like a better idea. I dragged a small Persian carpet from the living room floor out onto the deck. The warmth of the sun felt wonderful. I did a few gentle stretches. Freyja, curious, watched every move I made.

When I had finished stretching, I stood with my eyes closed, weaving to the music. I started moving my arms as if conducting an invisible orchestra. At first I concentrated on my normal side, willing my injured side to follow. My whole body started to move with the music.

The movement flowed naturally into dancing, releasing an energy I'd forgotten I had. My dancing was a sheer ignorance of physics, a sensation between my body and the air. I danced solo to the sun, gliding, drifting, letting the movement itself take control.

As if from another world, I heard Jenny's voice. "What are you doing?"

"What does it look like?"

"Dancing."

"Right."

She was silent for a moment and then she said, "Guess what I did?"

There was something about the tone of her voice that made me open my eyes. Her face looked rosy and healthy. "What?" I asked.

She smiled an exhausted, dreamy smile. "I just ran ten miles."

"You did what?"

"Yeah, it was a marathon. There were thousands of us. It was awesome, Mom."

Momentarily captured by the image, I contemplated what she had just said. I had run a few marathons myself, and knew how her body must feel.

I wrapped my arms around her. "Oh, my poor baby—you must hurt all over."

Her head pressed against my shoulder. I asked, "Why didn't you tell me you were doing this?"

"Well, I did, sort of … I said I was staying over at Jen's so that we could do a run in the morning."

"Jenny, until I'm back in the saddle, you're going to have to start treating me like someone with a head injury. You're going to have to look directly into my eyes and say: 'Earth to Mommy—do I have your attention?'"

She smiled. "All I want right now is a shower," she said. Like a sleepwalker, she dragged herself slowly up the stairs.

I pulled the carpet back to the living room, then picked up my research notes and went back out onto the deck to study. I nodded off, then I woke slowly, feeling I had lost the heat of the sun. I looked up at the sky and watched a cloud pass by in a great hurry.

I wondered about Jenny and went inside to find her. The shower wasn't on, so I pushed the bedroom door open a few inches. She was lying supine on her bed, her limbs flung out from her body. She had put on my white robe and wrapped a towel around her wet hair. Her mouth was open. I smiled and watched her for a few moments, then gently pulled a quilt over her and shut the door behind me.

Sunday was a beautiful spring day. Peter and I enjoyed a quiet breakfast together before he went off to finish his project. A very stiff-limbed Jenny headed out for a day of fun with her friends. Katherine came home from an early-morning shift at the restaurant and sat with me on the deck, sipping coffee and dozing in the welcome heat.

I breathed in the warmth of the air. Freyja kept wandering around us, and eventually she came and put her nose under my right arm, giving me a nudge. "Ouch," I said.

"Oh, no," Katherine moaned. "Freyja hasn't been walked yet."

"Not to worry, I'll do her," I offered. "You don't look like you want to move."

"I don't. It's all the standing and walking with this job. A lot of hungry people are just so unpleasant to deal with."

Freyja was on a tear, pulling me along like a water-skiier until I let her off lead. When we came back, the car was gone. I spotted a note by the telephone: "Mom, I'm out for a while. I'll call you. K."

I poured myself a cup of coffee. How strange, I thought; Katherine looked almost comatose when I left. Her note had obviously been written in great haste. My instincts told me that something was wrong.

I tried to do a little weeding, and then I carried the tele-phone outside and sat in a chair, waiting. When the phone rang, I grabbed it before it had even finished its first ring. "Hello?"

"Mom, I'm at the hospital. Jenny's okay—do you hear me? She's okay."

"Yes."

"But she's had a fall off her bike."

"How bad a fall?" I asked.

"She was knocked out—"

I took a big swallow. "Is she conscious?"

"Yes, but she doesn't remember the accident."

"I'll be right there."

"Mom, you can't drive."

"Oh, yes, I can."

"Mom, you don't even have a car."

"I'll find a ride—I'll call a taxi."

"Mom, will you listen to me for a minute? Jenny is okay. She's talking. She can even kind of smile."

"Where did it happen?"

There was a definite pause before Katherine answered. "At the canyon."

"The canyon," I shouted. "She's forbidden to bike at the canyon. No one in her right mind bikes at the canyon. Who was with her?"

"Tyler."

"Oh, Tyler," I groaned. Jenny and Tyler had been the best of friends since their first year in high school, and I liked him immensely. Katherine put him on the phone, and I asked him how it happened.

"We were going down this really steep bumpy part and I yelled at her to see if she was okay. She shouted back, 'Yeah, live and learn,' and then I heard this crash. I stopped and ran back. I had to follow the tire tracks to find her. She was just lying there—about twenty feet down the canyon—and she wasn't moving. I thought she was dead. Man, I just about flipped out because there was all this nothing right beneath her."

I had closed my eyes as Tyler told his story. She had been unconscious for several minutes, he said.

"What was she like when she came to?" I asked.

"Really confused at first. She kept saying over and over, 'What happened? What happened?' "

"She had her helmet on, didn't she?"

I heard the long pause and saved Tyler from having to answer. "The daughter of a paramedic out riding her bike without wearing a helmet?" I yelled into the receiver. I was mad now. It had long been a law in our family.

I closed my eyes again and tried to ground myself. After the run yesterday, couldn't she have given herself a day of rest?

There was silence on the line. When Katherine came back on I grilled her about Jenny's symptoms. Were there any other injuries? She told me that the hospital was X-raying a few areas, but the doctor thought Jenny probably just had a lot of scrapes and bruises.

"Okay, listen to me. I'm going to get myself in there just as fast as I can."

"Mom, it's crazy for you to come in. If the X-rays are okay, I can bring her home. The doctor told me to wake her up frequently in the night to check her because of the concussion."

That much I can handle, I thought to myself. "All right," I agreed. "I'll stay put if you promise to phone if there is any change."

"I promise."

I hung up the phone and held my head in my hands. I had lost control of my family. I had to get myself well again.

A humble and nauseated Jenny came home shortly afterwards. When I got over the shock of what her face looked like, I decided she was probably going to survive. There were no apparent fractures, although judging from the amount of swelling she had in her jaw, she was going to be in physiotherapy before I was.

I couldn't stop myself from asking the obvious question. "I want you to tell me one thing. Why no helmet?"

She put her hand up to her head as if she fully expected to find a helmet there. "I'm so sorry, Mom. I'd left my bike at Tyler's, but my helmet was in our car. I thought just once it wouldn't hurt—"

I kissed her forehead. She looked so pathetic. I put her in our bed, and she slept off and on for the rest of the day. I realized she had knocked one thing off my list of things to do. From the look of her, I wouldn't need to arrange rides to trumpet lessons for a few weeks.

When Peter got home, I filled him in on what had happened. "Why do you think she'd run in a marathon without training for it, and then the next day ride a bike at the canyon without wearing her helmet?"

He puffed thoughtfully on his pipe. "Perhaps it has something to do with her age—and with a nature that likes to jump now and see where she's landed after the fact."

"I normally feel I have an idea what she's doing and where she is—"

Peter looked at me. "Don't blame yourself. She's quite old enough to make her own decisions, and learn by them."

"I know that," I agreed. "It's just that I'm worried about the decisions she's making for herself right now."

Peter chewed thoughtfully on his pipe stem for a few

moments. "Should I sleep downstairs?" he asked. "I'm assuming you'll want to keep an eye on her."

"If you don't mind."

"I'll go get my things," he said, giving me a kiss.

Surprisingly, Jenny slept soundly despite my waking her every hour to check her pupils and level of consciousness. I didn't. I lay in the darkness listening for the sound of her breathing. It was a long night. The next day she had trouble opening her mouth wide enough for even a half-teaspoon. I fed her yoghurt, cut-up spaghetti, soup, Jell-O, applesauce, milk shakes—anything that might slip between her teeth. Outside the bedroom, some barn swallows had made a nest beneath the roof. We enjoyed watching the birds swoop busily in and out fetching tasty morsels for their babies.

While Jenny slept that afternoon, I played a few pieces on the piano. Today I was able to handle the Tchaikovsky piece without any difficulty. Now what to do about my legs, I wondered. I bent over from the waist like a Raggedy Ann doll and felt my muscles stretching. Then I climbed onto the exercise bike and started to peddle slowly. I was soon bored. I stopped and put on Albinoni's *Adagio for Guitar and Strings*. It had a dreamy quality, and it gave me the same wonderful feeling as soaring in a sail plane. As I paced myself to the music, I decided to throw in some visualization. I closed my eyes and envisioned my white cells racing through the circuits of my bloodstream gulping up all the bad cells. Then I thought of the army dune buggies silently crossing the deserts of Iraq. I imagined them accelerating through my veins, knocking out the enemy cells with their laser guns. I threw in a few "smart bombs" for any large tumours that might be lurking about and hoped there wouldn't be any collateral damage. Then, as I grew tired,

I imagined love flowing through my veins, healing everything it touched.

I stopped. To my delight, the digital read-out told me I had gone five miles. I was out of breath.

Jenny appeared on the stairs and said, "Do you think maybe you should call it a day, Mom?"

"Oh, but it felt so good." I grinned, the perspiration dripping from my forehead. I was pleased to see that other than looking like someone who had been hit by a car, Jenny was showing all the signs of getting back to normal.

For me, it was a relief to be doing something for someone else again. When Jenny wasn't needing attention, I busied myself at preparing the planters for flowers, sorting through the recycling bin and cooking a few meals. Surprisingly, it turned out to be a pleasant week for us at home. We were alone together most of the time.

Much to Jenny's disgust, I sent her back to school a week after the accident. She took a long time to get ready the first morning. She was obsessed with what she looked like. "What is everyone at school going to think when they see my face?"

"That's easy," I replied, grinning broadly. "They'll think, This is what a person looks like when she doesn't wear a helmet and she falls off a bike at the canyon. Cause and effect, my darling. You learned all about that when you were a baby."

Peter came downstairs and put his hand gently on my shoulder. "I think maybe we should leave that point alone now," he suggested. He slipped into his suit jacket and added with just a hint of a smile, "I think she's got the idea."

The moment they went out the door, I settled into a program of recovery with total and absolute determination. The pattern for the next two or three weeks was the same: wake up, have some coffee, eat breakfast, do exercises, conduct or dance to music, and then rest. I was soon conducting or dancing to Jenny's recording of Eric Clapton's *Unplugged* and the sound-track from *The Power of One*. After a shower, I'd find a spot of sun and do some studying. I'd fit in a few chores around the house and as many naps as I could. I even resorted to nosing the iron around a few shirts as a way of building up some strength in my right arm. I watched a ridiculous amount of television: it provided the mindless company I needed. I felt I should be swimming, but there was *that* problem with a bathing suit, and also the difficulty of transportation to the pool.

Before long I was able to walk to the beach, haul a kayak off the nearby boat rack and toss it into the ocean. But I was terribly discouraged to find that after about ten minutes I had to turn around and head for shore. I decided to stick to exercise where I wasn't constantly comparing my present capabilities with my former level of prowess.

Sundays rolled into Mondays and April turned into May. I walked for miles. Freyja was ecstatic with the new routine. When I got back from walking her, I'd have a rest and then ride my exercise bike for about a half hour; sometimes I closed my eyes and let my mind and body talk with each other. I imagined the cancerous cells growing smaller and smaller until they disappeared. I imagined my body becoming well and strong.

I had always wanted to cycle across France. I hung a map of the country on the wall beside the bike. I'd move a bright red pin along my route every time I completed ten miles. I started off in Calais and travelled through Paris with its mansard roofs and chestnut trees, its shutters opening to the spring light, its cob-blestoned streets. I imagined waving at Elaine, who might be sitting in a bit of sun at one of the little café tables. When I left Paris, I took a side trip through the Loire Valley, deciding that eventually I'd head into Pamploma for the running of the bulls.

Each day when I had a shower, I made my fingers crawl a tiny bit higher up the tiled wall. Eventually, I managed to raise my arm high enough to make it possible to shave underneath. I picked up a razor timidly. After one touch, I shrieked. Everyone, including Freyja, came rushing into the bathroom to see what had happened.

"Never," I shouted at them.

"Never what?" they asked in chorus.

"Never, as long as I live, will I shave under my arm. It felt just terrible."

Each of them let out a relieved sigh as they turned to leave.

When I came out of the shower, Peter was sitting in the bedroom chair taking off his shoes. He looked up at me. I had wrapped a towel around myself, sauna-fashion, but as usual it fell off almost immediately.

"I'm sure there's a way of getting this to work," I said as I bent to pick up the towel. "I just haven't figured it out yet."

Peter didn't say a word. I felt his eyes taking in all of me. I tried to appear casual as I slipped into my robe as quickly as I could.

I found ways to get to countless doctors' appointments, and I started physiotherapy. Since there was no bus service between the city and where we lived, I had to rely on others for rides. I hated feeling dependent but was resigned to making it an experience from which I could grow. Neighbours called regularly to see if I needed anything. Cheryl, who called every day, threatened me with my life if she were ever to see me in a taxi.

Eve, my physiotherapist, was aghast when she first saw my scar. I had gone to Eve for six months of treatment after a back injury. She knew my body. I told her about the exercise program I had established for myself, and she added a few exercises to strengthen my shoulder and arm. My visits with her were primarily for laser treatments to try to break down the scar tissue.

I looked forward to these appointments. I'd lie on my back while she gently moved the head of the laser over every inch of my scar. Several times she screwed up her face and complained, "It's attached to your chest wall. It's attached to everything, and it won't budge."

I admitted, "Sometimes I despair that I'll never get full range of motion back."

"Oh, if I know you, you will." She paused for a moment and looked directly at me. "I've never said this to you, but after that back injury you had, I didn't think you'd be able to work at your job again."

"It never occurred to me that I wouldn't get back. It was just a matter of when."

"And there you have it. So much of healing is a matter of having the right attitude, and hard work."

I felt the prickly sensation of the laser travelling over my skin. "Mind you," she went on, "you're lucky that your doctor sent you in when he did. I get women who have had a mastectomy months before and they literally have no use of the limb on the affected side."

"It's a pretty ugly scar, isn't it?" I said, knowing she'd be able to compare mine with others she'd seen.

"Yep," she agreed. "It looks like a farmer took a rake and hoe and had a good go at you."

"I was kind of hoping it might look like a bite mark," I said with a grin.

She laughed and then looked at me with raised eyebrows. "But you've still got your life, haven't you?" she said, nodding her head in answer to her own question.

Sometimes after one of my appointments I'd have someone drop me off at Pat's. Either Pat or someone in my family would see that I got home. Deirdre and I talked or saw each other almost every day. She often invited me over to her place for a change of scenery. We sipped wine and nibbled at smoked salmon while watching astounding sunsets. I was comforted by the feeling of warmth we again shared.

Inevitably, it came time to be fitted for a prosthesis. I was very nervous and had Jenny drop me off at the pharmacy. I ducked into the store after checking to see that no nurses, doctors or paramedics I knew had spotted me from the nearby hospital. I wanted total privacy on this mission.

The woman I had talked to previously was behind the counter. She greeted me as if we were old friends. Pulling a tape around her neck, she led me into a small fitting room. I lifted my arms out from my body as she placed the tape around my chest just beneath the breast area. She asked me to take a deep breath.

"My goodness," she said, "you must be a runner."

I smiled, deciding not to tell her my chest expansion had reached its present capacity because I conducted invisible orchestras, danced to my teen-aged daughter's music, and was riding an exercise bike across a map of France. She showed me a variety of bras and I tried them all to see which was the most comfortable. She selected a state-of-the-art prosthesis that best matched my left breast, and we both studied the finished picture in the mirror.

Next I tried on some bathing suits. I wanted one badly. A bathing suit told me symbolically that my life would continue to be active, as it had been before the surgery. I selected a suit I liked and was pleased with the way it looked.

"No one would ever know," the woman said, smiling. As discreetly as possible, she added, "A lot of women are a bit shy about making love at first. We often suggest a little camisole be worn." She waited for me to respond. When I didn't, she asked, "Would you like to try one?"

I turned to the task of getting my clothing back on and shook my head. "No, thank you." I wanted to get out of there fast.

I took my new breast home cradled in its special carrying case. The bill for everything had come to a staggering six hundred dollars. I decided to treat this new item with the utmost respect. For a week or two I did nothing but steal small looks at it from time to time. My prosthesis lay on one side of the bed at night while my husband lay on the other.

15

REGAINING THE ABILITY TO DRIVE gave me a whole new feeling of confidence and self-sufficiency. I visited people when I felt like it and left when I felt like it. I didn't have to ask for favours or worry about inconveniencing others. I phoned my professor and made arrangements to do my exam a few days later.

It was a warm sunny day out at the university, and the grass was littered with students studying, necking or just staring blankly at whoever walked by. I wrote the exam in the professor's office. I had no idea what my doctor had said in his letter, but my professor was kind and accommodating. I left the university knowing I had a safe pass, and that meant I would get my degree.

Back at home, I heated up some leftover coffee and sank into a deep leather chair with a couple of books. I had picked up Bernie Siegel's *Love, Medicine and Miracles* several times before, but each time I read a few pages I became slightly more horrified. *Getting Well Again*, by Carl Simonton, Stephanie Matthews-Simonton and James Creighton, had the same effect on me. Although both books were full of testimonials meant to make me feel that if I followed their teachings I might live another year—or five or ten—both linked the incidence of breast cancer to dysfunctional childhoods and mismanaged emotions later in adulthood. I didn't mind believing that positive thinking might help me get well, but I was reluctant to accept that I might have allowed the illness to happen. However, since I was determined to consider anything that might help me, I decided to tackle these two books today.

Siegel and the Simontons held that breast cancer could result from two different types of stress. The first was considered to occur on an unconscious level, as it originated in crippling childhood psychological trauma. The second type was more overt in nature—it stemmed from suffering a major loss, or from depriving the body and mind of proper relaxation, rest, exercise and emotional expression. Both kinds of stress were believed to inhibit the immune system, thereby allowing cell mutations to occur.

I had certainly experienced childhood trauma. I knew too that I lived a life busy enough to verge on careening out of control. Page by page, I became a little braver. After all, the body-mind concept was by no means new. The Romans believed that mind over matter—and mind over disease—was a reality. The idea that the mind had no role in creating serious illnesses came about with the new scientific understanding of disease.

I went into the kitchen, poured some coffee and watched steam rise from its black surface. I took a sip, left the mug on the counter, and went back to my chair.

Bernie Siegel, a cancer surgeon, maintained that the lives of breast cancer patients differed from patients with other types of cancer in an important way: breast cancer patients frequently had not had an opportunity to express their emotions as children. When an established relationship—or investment in a "significant other"—fell apart in adulthood, the original despair and hopelessness of the damaged inner child reemerged. The injured adult passively surrendered and thereby became vulnerable to disease.

Katherine's voice drifted into the study. "Whatever you are reading, I think you'd better stop. You look mad." She glanced at the Simontons' book, which she'd bought for me. "Oh," she said.

"They make it all sound so straightforward—your coping skills are shitty so you get cancer."

"I bought the book because I'd heard the emphasis was on helping people *fight* cancer."

"It is. It's just that I'm having trouble with their approach." I held the book in the air. "According to these people, I should consider cancer to be the best thing that ever happened to me—if it doesn't kill me—because now I am aware I must change my values, my lifestyle, my self-image ..."

"There might be something to it," she said hesitantly. "I mean, you *are* the most together woman I know on the face of this planet, but I also think there are some areas you could be working on."

"Like?"

"You're often stressed right out—"

"I'm not."

"You are. You do a tremendous job of not burdening anyone with it, but it's there."

I tossed the book into the wastepaper basket. "I know I'm a workaholic, but I love working. When I feel stressed by it I go kayaking or climb a mountain. I think I have good stress-coping skills."

Shaking her head, she retrieved the book, taking it with her into the kitchen. "What is this?" she demanded, picking up the glass coffee pot and gawking into it.

"Egg shells," I said. "The coffee was so strong I took some shells out of the compost. Makes the coffee taste better. Something your father taught me."

She put the pot back on the burner as if there were something dead inside it. Coming back empty-handed, she slumped into a chair beside me. "Speaking of stress," she said, "I've got to come up with something other than waitressing. I hate it. Hungry people are so miserable."

"Well, you were once interested in the ambulance service," I said.

"I still am."

"Then why don't you try the courses and see how it goes?"

"I'm a little short on the experience level. Don't most of the people hired have strong nursing or medical backgrounds?"

"I didn't, and I've done fine. You'd just have to work twice as hard as those who have experience. What's most important is a genuine caring for other people. And you certainly have that."

She studied me with silent concentration. "Go see if you can get into a course," I encouraged her. "It's difficult to get hired, but I've recently heard of a few openings. I think you'd make an excellent paramedic." I wrote down some names and phone numbers and told her where to start. She went off to make the calls.

In a few minutes she came back into the study, obviously pleased. "It's all set," she said. "I'm in a course at Trauma Tech next month."

"Congratulations," I said. "When you've finished that course, you can apply to the ambulance service. I hope I'm not introducing you to one of the most stressful jobs in the world."

"You don't find it that way."

"No, I love it. But the shift work is definitely not healthy. That I know for sure. My body frequently has no idea if it's day or night. I somehow doubt that going from sound asleep to full throttle is good for anyone either. And I guess it can get stressful when I try to fit so much more into my life at the same time."

"Waitressing is stressful," she said.

"Because you hate waitressing," I replied. "You know, from everything I've been reading, I can't help but wonder if breast cancer is partly due to not heeding what all mothers try to teach their children: 'If you don't look after yourself, you are going to get sick.' I'm sure it was originally intended to mean eating, sleeping and getting exercise. But all of that has been screwed up by the human population not looking after its world. We've turned our planet into a hostile place."

Despite her interest in environmental issues, I could see Katherine was no longer listening. I smiled, knowing that she was off somewhere chasing ambulances.

"Has anyone seen my boob?" became a frequently heard plea in our house. I swore that my prosthesis moved from place to place in the hands of an invisible mischief-maker several times a day. As it was still so uncomfortable to wear, I took it off at every opportunity: after coming in the front door, at my desk, after dinner. I finally gave up on the special bras sold by the prosthesis shop and thanked the heavens for my sports bras. The stretchable cotton was soft and didn't rub against my sore body. The bras had a fold of material at the bottom of the cup that conveniently held the prosthesis in place. But they weren't really made with this use in mind, so it was quite possible for the prosthesis to fall out while I was putting my bra on or taking it off. The sound it made as it hit the floor—like a soft grapefruit—became commonplace at home.

Eventually, I learned to remove the prosthesis only while I was getting dressed or undressed. That way I always knew where it was. It took me a while longer to get used to how cold the prosthesis was when I first put it on. If I had time, I'd hold it between my hands before slipping it into my bra, but frequently I just had to grin and bear it. If I was having a shower or bath, I'd sometimes throw the thing into the tub so that the water could warm it up.

All in all, this novelty piece had high entertainment value. I would make deals with my daughters: "If you get me some tea, I'll let you play with my boob." When it fell on the floor, Freyja would jump to attention and eye it fiercely. I was relieved her instincts somehow informed her not to attack.

The problem of not being able to wear a deodorant was not so easily solved. The skin under my right arm refused to tolerate the countless deodorants I tried. My environmentally aware daughter solved the problem by handing me a box of baking soda.

I was getting stronger and stronger. I made plans to return to work. I went back to Dr. Harris for another check-up.

"I'd like to see you again next week," he said at the end of the appointment.

"Actually, I'm busy next week," I told him.

"You fit me in whenever you can," he said. He smiled, and I knew he understood.

I returned to work on the first day of June, exactly two months from the date of my surgery. I was probably in better physical condition than I'd been in for many years, yet I was aware of the weakness in my right shoulder. Heavy lifting above shoulder height would be a challenge.

On the Saturday morning I started back, the air was bright and clear with purpose. I turned up at the station a little early so that I could check through the ambulance and go over paperwork that had appeared in my absence. Jeff and Brian, who had just worked a busy night shift, staggered out of the bedrooms to say hello. Dwayne, my partner for my first shift, said he'd already made sure the ambulance was clean and stocked.

Someone had put flowers on my desk, but no one would own up to the deed. There was also a cake with "Welcome Back" written in icing. I cut a piece for everyone, but we'd only taken one mouthful when we received our first call: "Routine for an unknown problem."

"Your choice, Roz—would you like to attend or drive?" Dwayne asked.

"I'll attend if you don't mind," I said. I had missed the contact with patients.

A very young police officer met us outside the house. He didn't seem to know much except that a young woman had lived here by herself for about a year and a concerned neighbour had contacted the police. As we walked through the front door, the scene was so dramatic that it was like being dropped into someone else's dream. Everything in the small house had been crudely painted with wild strokes of blue: floors, ceilings, furniture, a rolled carpet, dishes, appliances, light fixtures, even the windows.

I could hear a woman talking in one of the rooms. I asked the officer, "Do you know her name?"

The young rookie was trying to take in every angle at once. "No," he said. "The neighbours say she keeps to herself."

I bent over and picked up some unopened mail lying on the floor. Several envelopes showed her first name as Sara. I handed the mail to the officer and moved towards the voice.

As I entered the dining room, I saw the woman in a mirror. She was standing at the window. The early morning sun forcing its way through the painted glass gave the room a strange quality. The bottom of the mirror had been left unpainted, but narrow trickles of paint had hardened on its surface. In between the blue streaks were flesh tones. The woman was naked.

I waited until my eyes had adjusted to her blue-lit world, then slowly walked up to her. I heard her say, "How many are there? I don't know. What do they matter? I have no idea."

I spoke softly. "Sara, my name's Rosalind. I'm with the ambulance service."

She didn't look at me, but she said, "The night protects your face."

"Sara, are you in pain?"

"We go where they go, no one knows, no one knows ..."

I guessed her to be in her late twenties. There were no obvious signs of injury or illness. I thought of Picasso's blue period. He had found blue a screen behind which he felt secure. But he had also seen blue as sadness and death, loneliness and the absence of love. What was blue to Sara? Was it sky? There were areas where the bold blue strokes looked like waves. Was it water? Dreams? Memories? Something else entirely?

"Sara, could you sit down and talk to me?"

She didn't take her eyes away from the blue window. "There's no way to know. No way at all."

I motioned for Dwayne to bring the stretcher close by. I pulled the blanket off the top and wrapped it around her shoulders.

"Sara, we are going to take you to the hospital. Can you sit on the stretcher for us?"

"We go where they go."

I gently eased her back onto the stretcher. There was no resistance, but she had closed her eyes. Her face had a stony, masklike quality. As we wheeled her from the otherworldliness of her house to the ambulance, I heard her say, "We go with the hoofprint in the sky of blue."

I glanced at the neighbours' houses and saw faces in nearly every window. I knew I was back at work.

16

HAVING FINISHED FOUR BUSY DAYS in a row at work, I sat and relaxed in front of the television. My last two shifts had been night shifts, and my biological time clock was all mixed up again. I hadn't been able to sleep during the day, so watching television seemed about the right speed for me. Everyone else in the family was away until the next day, so I had the house to myself.

I clicked the channel selector several times and settled on a late-night news special summarizing everything of significance that had happened in the world so far that year. It filled in some blocks of time I had missed while I was in hospital or too distracted to assimilate the information. Many of the news items brought back feelings I'd experienced at the time of the events.

The focus was still on the Gulf War. I thought it strange that I couldn't remember the exact moment when the war had been declared over. I watched a British tank flying the skull and crossbones as it manoeuvred slowly along the road to Basra, which had been bombed by Allied aircraft. The men from the Royal Engineers called themselves the graves commission; their job was to bury the dead and clear the wreckage from the highway.

I saw more footage of Hussein's scorched earth campaign; a journalist referred to it as "a nuclear winter." A moot point, I reflected, that the war was over. Shots of camels mesmerized by a horizon of fire were reminiscent of Dante's vision of hell.

I felt a soreness in my left breast and put my hand up to gently massage it. There were shots of soldiers dragging other soldiers away. I listened to the reporter call the actions of the victors "a witch-hunt." He expressed alarm that there was little to distinguish these actions from the actions of the Iraqis.

My fingers returned to something I had felt in my breast. A western diplomat was being interviewed. He said that America should become the "globo-cop" and police the world against small-time dictators. I took my hand away, then felt my breast again and said, "No." There was a close-up of President Bush. He was addressing Congress. The Gulf War was the "first test of a new world coming into view, a world in which there is the very real prospect of a new world order," he said. The commentators interpreted this message as meaning a world order in which the superpower struggle had ended and nasty dictators did what they were told by the United States. They quoted Bush's 1988 nomination acceptance speech: "We saved Europe, cured polio, went to the moon and lit the world with our culture."

I sat on the edge of the sofa. I felt hot and weak. Over and over I felt a lump low down in my left breast, and again and again I said, "No, it isn't there." I stared unseeing at the blur of the television screen. After a time I got up and switched it off. I had a momentary sensation of weightlessness. I caught my breath. I didn't know what to do with myself; I started wandering from room to room, picking things up and putting them down again. Freyja watched attentively as I went from one level of the house to the next.

A vague sensation of being hunted propelled me back to the sofa. I stared at the blank gape of the television screen for a long time. Once again I feared something I could feel but not see.

The phone rang, startling me. I looked at it until the answering machine clicked on. No one spoke. The machine beeped, and then there was nothing but silence.

My hands shook. What had I just heard on television—that the United States had voted an emergency $2 billion for weapons? How many more billions were pumped into the military? I remembered reading reports of President Nixon's promise twenty years ago to make finding "the magic bullet"— the cure for cancer—a priority. Twenty years ago, it had been projected that one in four Americans would contract cancer during his or her lifetime. Now it was one in three, and breast cancer was leading the epidemic.

I leaned my head back against the wall. I thought of a newspaper clipping pinned to the wall of my study. It was a story about a $100-a-plate fund-raiser for breast cancer, in

Toronto. The reporter wrote that a person could "go ballistic" when looking at the almost nonexistent dollars for breast cancer research in Canada. In the current year the bean counters in Ottawa were spending $14 million on AIDS research. The point of the article was that the number of women in Canada who would die from breast cancer in that year was almost twice the total number of AIDS deaths in the country since 1979. Something was seriously wrong here. AIDS research had started to receive the money it deserved. Why hadn't breast cancer?

I got up and switched on the fan over the stairs to cool down the house. I put my hand on the telephone and then thought: Nobody is going to want to hear about this. I tried to pretend the lump wasn't there, but each time I felt my breast the world came crashing in on me. I had a terrible sense of déjà vu.

I lay in bed listening to the fan clicking against the silence. The noise stopped for a moment, and I found myself holding my breath. I started breathing again only when the reassuring, inconsequential sound of the ticking resumed. I was exhausted, but I couldn't sleep. I got up and restlessly prowled the house. I tried a bath. A glass of milk. A few pages of reading. Nothing worked. Finally I went back to bed. I spent the night tossing and turning.

In the morning, I phoned to make an appointment with Dr. Harris. I sounded very calm as I explained to the nurse that I might have a mass in my other breast. She told me she'd had a cancellation and I could come in right away. I threw on yesterday's jeans and a clean shirt and set out for his office.

The very act of stepping into the elevator of the medical building turned my stomach. I gazed in resignation at the familiar walls of Dr. Harris's waiting room. It was full of new faces. I had the feeling that the nurse had fit not only me but many other women into an already busy day. I was surprised at how quickly my name was called.

Dr. Harris said it was good to see me. I asked him to check my left breast and wondered if the nurse had said anything to him about what I had found. Smiling slightly, I told him, "You have to give that breast twice as much time now that I have only one."

Despite his busy morning, he didn't make me feel hurried. His hand methodically palpated my breast. He stopped to the left of my sternum—just where I had felt the lump.

I watched his face. I got the feeling that he didn't like what he had found. While he carefully pressed on the breast tissue, he asked, "How long is it since I've checked this breast?"

"A month maybe?"

He asked me to sit up and move my arms first out from my body and then up over my head. I knew he was looking for puckering or dimpling, signs of malignancy.

"That looks okay," he said, stroking his chin with his hand. His eyes met mine. "It's a concern, isn't it?"

I nodded. "What do you think?"

He inhaled, then made a strange whistling sound through his teeth as he let the air out. "Whatever it is, it's very hard."

He thought for another moment or two and then pulled out a pair of sterile gloves. "I'm going to try a needle aspiration and see what happens."

I drew in a quiet breath, watching. As before, the needle aspiration was unsuccessful. I let out a small sigh. "When it works, women must think you're the greatest doctor in the world."

He didn't smile. "Well—"

"Well?"

"It's back to the question of where we go from here. What do you want to do?"

"I want to know what it is."

He nodded his head. "It's not loose like we'd expect of a malignant tumour. It seems to be attached to your chest."

"I know someone who recently died in palliative care because she had a lump attached to her chest and her doctor didn't think it was anything to worry about."

"Yes, you've mentioned her to me. That's one of the problems with breast cancer. There's not much we know for sure."

I smiled a little. "I've been learning that," I said.

He flipped through the pages of my file. "My advice has always been that if a woman feels there is something wrong with a lump she should insist on a biopsy. Not everyone agrees with me. But the way I look at it—if she's wrong, it'll put her mind at rest. If she's right, she just may save her own life."

"Does this mean more surgery?"

"Not what you need right now, is it?"

I shook my head, wondering why I hadn't prepared myself for this.

"Maybe we'll have cells from this needle biopsy that will give us some information. But the lump is there and you don't want it there—right?"

"Give me your professional opinion. Am I overreacting? Should I just be keeping an eye on it?"

"You're not overreacting. With something like this, even with a negative finding, we'd still want to follow it up with a surgical biopsy." He closed his eyes tightly and then opened them again. He looked as if he hadn't had any more sleep than I'd had. "There's another difficulty at the moment. I leave tomorrow for a two-week holiday."

I remained dead silent.

He leaned back on the stool. "It isn't jeopardizing your situation to wait two weeks for an excisional biopsy, but you may not want to because of the worry. If you'd like, I can refer you to another doctor who could do the biopsy for you. He may be able to get you into the hospital before I can."

I heard myself answer, "I'll wait until you get back."

The small room hummed with silence. Dr. Harris sat looking at me and then gave me a tired smile. "I'll have Nancy book a time right away so that the surgery can happen immediately upon my return. It's going to be a busy time when I get back. It's frightening how many women are walking into this office right now." He gazed out the window for a moment and then looked back at me. "I'll also request one of the anaesthetists on the list you gave me. It will be the same two-step procedure as last time. We'll do a frozen section of the lump at the time of surgery. If we find a malignancy, we'll remove a margin of breast tissue around the area of the tumour but nothing more. Then we'll wait for the lab results before discussing the next step. Any questions?"

I shook my head and tried to make light conversation. "Are you going anywhere interesting for your holidays?"

He broke into a grin. "I'm going fishing. I have a friend who has a troller, and each year I help him with his catch for a couple of weeks."

I smiled. "Take care of your hands, won't you?"

Not for the first time, I left his office feeling numb. As I drove home, I remembered reading about a doctor who routinely biopsied the second breast in the same area if he found a malignancy in the first.

I reminded myself that so far everything had more or less worked out for me. But I knew that for some women things didn't work out. I knew that if my cancer had spread, it might soon kill me.

I stopped on the way home to go for a walk along the ocean. I had fleeting visions of faraway seas I wanted to visit, experiences I had yet to have, books I had yet to write. My eyes shifted to the blue sky, and I thought that somehow, somewhere up there, there had been a serious miscalculation. I picked a flower from a clump of daisies and carried it down to the rocks, where I sat listening to the repetitive sound of the waves. Slowly, I pulled off the petals of the flower one by one: "Live, die, live, die, live, die ... live, live."

That evening was one of the rare occasions when everyone happened to be home at the same time. I looked at the people I loved sitting around the dining room table, and it occurred to me again that it was not one traumatic experience or another that wore a person down, but the moments in between.

I drew in my breath sharply and decided on the direct approach. "Listen, I have this little lump in my left breast that I'm having biopsied in a couple of weeks."

There wasn't a sound. As I sliced a piece of melon, I knew every eye was on me. I didn't know what else to say. Strangely, what I thought about was that, at this very moment, other women very like me and yet very different were speaking these same words to their families.

"What are you saying?" Katherine asked finally, wiping her hands on her apron.

"I have another lump. It's probably nothing. But it needs to be removed."

"Is this something you've just discovered?" Peter's voice was quiet, calm.

"Yes. Actually, I felt it yesterday and went to the doctor today. He's going away for two weeks so he's going to remove it when he gets back."

I looked over at Jenny. She had grown perceptibly smaller in her chair. We all sat motionless, lost in the information, as if time had finally caught up with us.

It was a hot summer night. I lay on my side and watched Peter get ready for bed. I could hear the ceiling fan slowly turning. He switched off the light and crawled under the sheet beside me. In the faint illumination from the window I could tell he was looking at me.

"I'm so sorry this has happened to you," he said.

"It may be nothing."

"You've already gone through so much ... I wish there was something I could do."

He ran one of his hands slowly down my back. I shuddered and pulled away. Gently, he drew me back towards him. He put his arms around me. Except for our breathing, we stayed still for the longest time. I felt a warmth spreading through me. He kissed me, and I kissed him back, deeply. I let his nakedness move slowly against me until my body answered. With the anticipation of beginners, we moved slowly, like swimmers in a dream.

It was morning. The bed was still warm from Peter's body, and I could hear him in the shower. I stretched, feeling the last wave of the pleasure that had awakened me from my deep sleep.

I got up and took a cup of coffee out into the forest to drink it in the sunshine. I watched some wasps making a paper house in a tree. When Peter was ready to leave, he came out and joined me for a few minutes.

"Do you have any plans for today?" he asked.

"Just to enjoy *being*," I said. "Oh, I'm also taking Deirdre out for a late birthday lunch."

"Good," he said. He wrapped his arms around me. Jenny popped her head out the front door, asking if I'd iron her a shirt for work.

"Can't you see I'm busy?" I said, grinning.

"Well, you guys can't do that forever."

"Oh, yes we can." Peter kissed me, and I watched until he had gone down the stairs to his car.

After Katherine and Jenny left for the day, I had a shower, then walked Freyja to the waterfall. I sat watching the rainbow in the spray of water above the falls while I tried to organize my thoughts. Freyja was exploring, but she kept running back to me with an intense expression. Usually I envied her for being oblivious, but today, when I looked at her eyes, I wondered how much she was aware of. As we climbed the hill to go home the promise of another hot day filled the air.

I needed to find out what the possibility of cancer in my second breast meant. I pulled out *Dr. Susan Love's Breast Book.* The book opened to a line that caught my attention: "Women don't give themselves breast cancer, and they won't help themselves by feeling guilty about something they didn't bring on themselves." I read on. Dr. Love agreed that stress could depress the immune system and that women with a fighting spirit appeared to have a somewhat better survival rate than "passive victims." Yet she was also appalled by a study that indicated "41 per cent of women with breast cancer think they brought it on themselves because of the stress in their lives."

I flicked over a few more pages and stared at a diagram of a tumour travelling from a woman's breast to her lungs and liver. It gave me the creeps. I read that the average cancer has a doubling time of approximately one hundred days. I considered the size of my lump and quickly calculated that before surgery I housed almost 3 billion cancer cells. What were the chances, I wondered, that a few of those hadn't hit my bloodstream? According to Dr. Love, I would have to depend on my immune system to kill off the roving cells.

I decided to quit scaring myself to death and got back to looking for the information I wanted. I found it under "Second

Primary." Dr. Love wrote that, although it happens, it's rare for a breast cancer to metastasize from one breast to another. Usually cancer in a second breast isn't a recurrence but a separate new cancer. On the down side, this suggested that for whatever reason a patient's breast tissue was prone to developing cancer. On the up side, a patient's prognosis was "as bad as the worst of your two cancers." I chose to consider this good news. I knew that what I had just read was about as good as it got with this disease—choices between negatives. There might not be much room for certainty, but there was room for optimism.

Dr. Love believed a woman was wise to think of breast cancer as a chronic disease, but she added, "In retrospect, if you're dying of something else at a ripe old age, you will know that you were also wise if you thought of it as something you can live with."

I tossed the book aside. The lines of an old cowboy song that Peter liked to sing came to mind: "If the hard times don't kill me, I'll live till I die …"

I looked at my watch and decided it was time to get ready to meet Deirdre. Feeling the heat rising, I was glad we had decided on a restaurant where we could eat outside under an umbrella and watch the nearby waves roll onto the shore.

When I arrived, Deirdre already had a drink, and she was facing the ocean. I could tell by her expression that she was off somewhere. I'd always enjoyed observing her when she thought she was alone; that was when she seemed most herself.

Baroque music was playing in the background. I rounded the table. A look of delight transformed her face as I sat down opposite her.

"So, what kept you?" She grinned. She was usually the one who was late.

She put her sunglasses on. She looked terrific, but I had always thought of her as hiding behind those glasses.

She said, "You look wonderful with that tan."

"I feel great."

"How's work going?"

"Let's see," I said, chewing on a crust of bread. "Last shift, we had a baby around midnight; we got a bone caught in our throat around 3:00 A.M.; about an hour later, we had a heart attack and drove a car into a tree."

"Did we die?"

"Briefly."

We laughed. I pushed a pat of butter around a small plate with my knife.

"You writing these days?" she asked.

"Not really." My drink arrived and I swilled it down, asking the waiter for a large glass of water. "I've been pretty busy— back at work, boning up on my protocols and what have you."

We sat talking about one thing or another until I realized how hungry I was. We ate slowly, savouring each mouthful.

"What do you order after a lunch like that?" I asked.

"Brandy," she said. "But I'd better pass. I have to drive home."

We drank coffee, chatting while the deepening sun crossed the sky. Time always passed too quickly when we were together.

"Thursday, can you do lunch?" she asked, getting up from her chair. "Potluck—at my place?"

I shook my head, genuinely disappointed. "I work day shift."

The sun flashed off her dangly silver earrings. "No problem," she said. "We'll start lunch late in the afternoon."

"I can probably get early coverage," I offered.

"Wonderful. I'll tell the others to come around five."

"What can I bring?"

"Nothing."

"If it's potluck, I want to bring something."

"Bring wine then." She waited while I pushed my chair away from the table. "We never seem to have too much wine." She laughed.

The morning of the potluck I woke up feeling a sharp but undefined sadness. Maybe it was because the discomfort left over from my surgery had seemed particularly wearing these last few days. Maybe it was the thought of what might lie ahead.

It was a tough day at work, too. A late call kept me from getting off work as early as I had hoped. The call was for an accident involving five cars. The patients weren't badly injured, there were just a lot of them. Liz Berry's husband was the attending police officer. We smiled to acknowledge each other but didn't talk. I wanted to ask him about his wife, but we were far too busy. And I feared his answer.

Even though I was already late for Deirdre's, I decided I wasn't going anywhere until I'd had a shower. I tried to blame the heat for my *down* day. Everything seemed such an effort. I climbed into an off-white cotton pantsuit with a permanent wrinkled look and put on my wooden beads so everyone would know I had dressed up.

Afternoon had become evening by the time I arrived at Deirdre's. I was surprised to see so many cars parked along the street. There were a few abstainers in our group of friends, so we had some ready-made designated drivers. We'd come up with a strategy of leaving a hat for keys just inside the front door. The drinkers were expected to walk home or arrange for a ride.

The door to Deirdre's house was ajar, and from the noise level I guessed that a lot of the cars would still be there in the morning. Pat pulled the door wide open with an exaggerated bow before I had even made it to the entrance. She had a beatific smile on her face. "Do you like wakes?" she said.

"I prefer Kahlúa and milk," I answered, my eyes trying to take in the scene behind her. She handed me a tall glass, already poured.

Before following Deirdre into the house, I dropped my keys into the hat. On a white linen tablecloth, tapers flickered in gold candlestick holders. There was an incredible spread of food. I stared at the centrepiece as I gulped down my Kahlúa. It was a sculpture of the Virgin with a rosary draped over her. Everyone else was drinking champagne. I was the only one not dressed in black.

"It's a wake," Pat said, walking through the crowd to fill my glass.

"A wake?" I asked, confused.

"It's a party," said Marcia cheerfully.

"Well then," I said, "let's get on with it." I raised my glass to them all and took another long drink.

Donna came up to give me a hug. She announced to the room, "I don't know if anyone else is as hungry as I am, but as far as I'm concerned, 'Let's get on with it' means 'Let's eat.'"

There was a round of cheers and applause. Slowly overcoming my bewilderment, I said, "I'm sorry. I had no idea."

"Not a problem," Marilyn said, closing in on me. "We've shown many times over the years that we didn't need the guest of honour to be present for us to have a good time."

I allowed a slightly wounded look to cross my face. Before I had a chance to notice that my glass was empty, it was taken from my hand and replaced by another.

After dinner, Deirdre produced a vial not much larger than her thumb. "Okay, everyone." She waved the bottle in the air. "What's a wake without snuff?"

I watched Pat roll eyes that said a catastrophe lay ahead. We experimented with the snuff, breaking into fits of laughter as the bottle was passed from hand to hand. Eventually it made its way to me. Following what the others had done, I made a little depression between my thumb and forefinger, dropped a bit of snuff there, and inhaled it through my nostrils. We sat holding our sides from the pain of laughing, none of us having any idea what we were laughing about.

With tears streaming down her face, Pat was the first to try to restore order. She tossed a wine cork high into the air. We all watched as it came down to nest deep in her cleavage.

She winked at me. "Like to see you do that, my sweet," she said. In the darkness of the room I noticed her reach for something that looked like a tall willow branch. Pencils, erasers, pens, notepaper and miniature bottles of Kahlúa hung from its bare boughs. "From us to you," she said. "The tree of life." She put her arm around me and lifted her drink in a toast:

> Drink on, drink on, my many friends all
> Feast on your food and your wine,
> For whatever is dealt at *her* wake today
> Shall be dealt tomorrow at mine.

There was thunderous applause. Pat planted the heavily laden branch in a boot and leaned it against the wall. I didn't have any idea what to say. I had caught the odd fleeting glance at my bosom, so I put my hand into my bra and pulled out my boob. I held it up for all to see, then told them how much it had cost. Amid many "oohs" and "aahs" it was passed reverently around the room until it ended up with me again.

The day's heat was still in the air. I watched a candle flame lean this way and that, wavering, recovering, swelling, like something alive. In the background I could hear Eric Clapton's *Unplugged*. The singer was well into "Tears in Heaven." My body started to move with an impulsive certainty. I stood up and started to do a few steps.

I heard Pat shout, "Oh, yes!"

I danced into the middle of the room. Moonlight flooded in through the window. I let the music flow through my body and possess me. When the tune was over, Marcia let out a whoop and demanded that I dance the next song. I understood that this party was meant to serve as a formal declaration of my recovery, and I allowed that spirit to carry me. Soon everyone was up on their feet, dancing. As they were all dressed in black, I could see only the candlelight flickering on their faces. Then I looked up at the ceiling. Looming over us were our shadows, moving as if controlled by the light of the moon. As though part of a dream, I moved in and out of the shadows, watching the images dance.

The others sat down as they tired. Before long, I was the only one left dancing. Fearlessly, I danced on. Someone put the same album on again and again, and the songs kept following each other. I broke into a sweat. Every so often a drink would be put to my mouth so that I could continue. It was as if there were another woman inside me dancing. I danced like a person with no past, no future and no other present but this moment. My energies, my life, surged through my body. How marvellous it felt to dance out the pain. Dancing, I was in control, invulnerable.

"Four hours," they announced in disbelief, as we congregated at the door to leave. "You danced for more than four hours!"

Away from the music, the street seemed absolutely silent. I walked home smiling, satisfied.

The next morning I walked over to Deirdre's to see if I could help her clean up the remains of the party. Her door was open when I arrived, and I shouted into what seemed to be an empty house. "Deirdre, are you home?"

"Good morning," she said, coming around the corner. I was relieved that she seemed pleased to see me. "Boy, you sure didn't fall asleep at last night's party."

I grinned back. "I'll remember that night of dancing as long as I live."

"So will we all." She laughed. "How is your body making out today?"

"A little stiff and sore," I admitted. "But I had expected worse."

"When I got up this morning, I looked to see if you'd worn a hole through the floor."

"No damage, I hope."

She shook her head, amused.

"Last night we were into pagan practices," I said, surprised to see such a tidy house. "I came over to see if I could help clean up."

"All done—but come in. Let's have coffee."

As we walked through the house, Deirdre's youngest daughter, who was two years younger than Jenny, came out of the kitchen. "What happened to you?" I asked, noticing bruises.

"Oh, I fell off my bike," she said.

"Not you too."

Deirdre was drumming her fingers on the kitchen counter. "Tell Rosalind the rest of the story."

"Well," she said, reluctantly, "I didn't have a helmet on."

"Oh, oh."

"I know," she said, looking back at her mother. "The stuff has already hit the fan around here about that." She started to climb the stairs to escape any more lectures.

"She didn't break anything, by the looks of it," I commented.

"No, but she has a concussion and a whopping headache."

"When did it happen?"

"Day before yesterday."

"You mean she was home in bed all during that party?"

"Yes."

"Poor girl—there's probably more than one reason she has a headache."

"Must be a run on bike accidents," Deirdre suggested.

"Don't laugh. It happens all the time at work. One day everyone who has ever considered having a stroke has one. Another day it will be asthma or chain saw accidents or aneurysms." I glanced at her in her black shorts and shirt, and added, "Like your father. How are you handling all of that now?" I asked gently.

"Oh, you know me—fine, fine, fine," she answered with a mock grin. She showed me some silverware and family photographs she had brought home from her father's place.

"Deirdre, how long do you have to keep going through all this stuff?"

"The worst of it is over. My oldest sister is coming into town tomorrow so we can finish the job." She shivered.

"Have you ever heard of the merits of ripping a band-aid off quickly?"

"I know. It's taken a lot out of me."

"I'm sorry you've had all of this to deal with. I haven't been much use to you, have I?"

"Not to worry. There's not much you could have done."

She poured two cups of coffee, and we took them out to a pair of rattan chairs that sat in a sunlit corner on her shadowed lawn. Under the kitchen window there was a wall of sweet peas. A handful of the flowers, in a profusion of colours, sat in a vase on a table beside me. I leaned over to smell their sweet fragrance.

"You know, I was just a little nervous about having a wake," Deirdre said. "Pat thought it was a great idea—but you know Pat." She glanced at me. "Were you okay with it?"

"I must confess, it threw me a little at first, but just momentarily. In case you didn't notice, I had a good time."

I took a sip of the hot coffee. "The problem I've been having … is on my mind a little more now than it might otherwise be. You know how we were talking about there being runs on things?"

We regarded each other for a moment.

"I seem to be having a run on breast lumps. There's one in my other breast. It's going to be biopsied next week."

"Oh, no," she moaned. "What timing for a wake." She put her hand on mine and gave me a look I couldn't interpret. Our eyes locked for a moment.

I leaned back and looked out at the ocean. "I wasn't going to tell you. But then I decided I'd be really angry if the situation were reversed and you didn't tell me."

I felt her watching me. "Rosalind, you've *done* all that. You're supposed to be moving on to new things now."

"I know."

She leaned towards me. "What do they think it is?"

I watched a monarch butterfly flit by my chair, half carried by a light breeze coming down the mountain. "Don't know," I told her. "That's why it has to go."

She sat back in her chair, seemingly preoccupied.

"I know I'll make it through all of this," I said to change the mood, "because I couldn't stand to miss one of our parties."

"They're getting stranger and stranger, aren't they?"

"Perhaps *we* are." I smiled at her. "Anyway, if you wouldn't mind keeping it quiet. Apart from my family, I've decided I'm only telling you and Pat. If other people hear about it they might write me off. I haven't written myself off, and I don't want anyone else doing it."

"Of course," she said.

The butterfly came back and landed on the toe of her sandal. We stared at it as if we were in a trance.

I went to bed that night before anyone else got home. Whenever it was warm, I liked to sleep with the windows and deck door open. As I lay there, I listened to a gentle wind carry the sound of the waves back into the mountains.

17

I CALLED PAT THE NEXT DAY. I told her I was considering the pending surgery as nothing more than an inconvenience. She asked me to come by for a visit.

She greeted me at the door in a flowered muumuu. I felt I was in the centre of a moving garden as she fussed over me. Before I left, she filled my arms with enough containers of tasty food to last my family a week.

"Remember those angels I sent down Howe Sound?" she said. "Well, they love being with you. Let's face it, they love Lions Bay. But just so you know, they're here for as long as you need them."

"Thanks, Pat," I said, loading the car. As I turned the engine over, I scanned the horizon, half-expecting a crowd of angels to appear and ferry me home.

The night before the surgery I was scheduled to work. I had tried to sleep during the day, but eventually I'd given up.

It was my turn to drive. My partner, Ken, checked out the ambulance. I called our dispatcher to let him know the night crew was now on duty. He told us things were frantic in the city and asked us to head in that direction.

It was a hot, sticky night in July. We weren't surprised that the city was busy. Heat does something to people. There was a lunar eclipse that night as well. Ken and I chatted, but I said nothing about my surgery the next morning.

When we got downtown, we responded to several routine calls. It was a night for emotional upsets and domestic disputes. We spent as much time as we dared in trying to settle people, transporting only two of them to hospital for further observation or treatment.

The pattern was broken by a call to a stabbing at one of the hotels in the heart of the city. All other ambulances in the area were busy, so we had no back-up. We were told not to enter the hotel without the police. Ken and I groaned, both familiar with the address. It was a crumbling relic with no elevator. The room number was 55. That meant we had to hike up five flights of stairs and then probably carry someone all the way down.

When we arrived at the call, a police car was parked at the scene. Leaving our warning lights blinking, we gloved up, grabbed our gear, and locked the doors of the ambulance behind us. We walked towards a waving flashlight to join the officer at the door.

"No power," he warned us.

In almost total darkness, we tailed the officer up the narrow stairway, following a trail of blood. From the way it had hit the stairs, we deduced that someone who was bleeding had left the building recently. With a little luck, I thought, it will be our patient, and we won't have to carry him down. I heard the officer call for back-up on his radio.

Our eyes slowly began to adjust to the darkness. People occasionally opened their doors to watch with dazed expressions as we went by, stumbling over garbage and empty liquor bottles. I felt their eyes on my back. When we reached the fifth floor, someone very drunk directed us to a door. The officer asked what had happened, but the drunk only weaved a little as he backed away and let out a string of obscenities.

Ken and I stood away from the door as the officer reached out sideways to knock and identify us to whoever was inside. We stayed clear, so that if anyone shot through the door, the shots would miss us. There was only a quiet moaning in the room. The officer tried the door handle, but it had been locked from the inside. He stepped back, then with one quick blur of his boot kicked in the door.

His flashlight scanned the room. Before long, the beam illuminated a figure lying in the middle of an uncovered mattress. The filthy bed was soaked in blood. The lights and noise of the world outside flooded in through the open window. Cars passing in the street dragged tall distorted rectangles of light across the opposite wall.

While Ken assessed our patient, I readied the equipment I thought he might need. I positioned myself so that my back was against the wall. From where I was standing, I could watch anyone who might enter the room and also keep an eye on Ken's back while he worked on the patient.

Ken confirmed that we had a stabbing and said that as soon

as he had the bleeding under control he wanted to move the patient—fast. I was only too happy to get out of there. I called dispatch on our portable radio and requested assistance in carrying our patient out to the ambulance.

I listened to the officer's voice in the hall. He was shouting now in his attempt to determine what had happened. For the most part I ignored the litany of curses that he received in answer. I knew that he was even more used to it than I was, but I was also aware that the emotions that had precipitated the stabbing were still running strong. Then I heard someone swearing just outside the door. A drunk weaved in with such a sense of belonging that I wondered if we were in his room.

"What the fuck took you so long?" he shouted at us. Almost simultaneously the officer appeared and pushed the staggering derelict against the wall. Still the obscenities flowed. The officer rough-armed him out the door.

I took a last quick look around for any identification or medications that might give us some information about our patient. I found nothing. I noticed a pair of trousers under the bed. I carefully checked the pockets. Nothing. There didn't appear to be any evidence of drug abuse, either. Just beer and whiskey bottles everywhere.

I shouted to the officer, "Ask our friend who this guy is—I can't find any I.D."

An answer was shouted back. "He says he doesn't know."

"I bet," I said quietly to Ken, who had glanced up at me.

We started the long hike down the stairs with our John Doe securely fastened to the stretcher. It was rough going because of the weight of the patient and the challenge of finding our footing in the darkness. We had to lift the stretcher over newel posts at each turn of the stairs. My right shoulder was screaming with the carry. I tried to ignore it and let my adrenalin pick up some of the load, hanging on until a fire crew met us halfway down.

When the street air hit me, I knew I'd worked up a good sweat. A few lost souls loomed around us as we lifted our patient into the back of the ambulance. On went the lights and siren. We wove in and out of cars, buses, taxis and pedestrians. It was not yet midnight, and this shift had all the makings of one that would never end.

As soon as we were clear of the hospital, Ken and I cruised the city streets, discussing our John Doe, waiting for the next call. It was only a matter of minutes until we were sent to a nearby address for a "jumper." We parked the ambulance, and as we approached, a witness told us that someone had jumped from the roof. We looked up. The building must have been at least twenty floors high.

As we moved in on our patient, the bystanders gave us a wide, respectful berth. A quick assessment told us there was nothing to be done. I guessed the young male had been in his twenties. His body appeared muscular, and he had probably been in pretty good physical shape. What really bothered me was that the patient's head, still on his body, was twisted backwards, facing the opposite direction. Heads were not supposed to do that. From long ago, a feeling came back to me. For an instant, I was a child staring at the twisted body of my father. We put a blanket over the young man, leaving the body for the coroner. I took a last long look and felt an involuntary shudder. He had worn a tux, and I wondered why. What had his last thoughts been? Who might be expecting him home?

I drove slowly down the busy night streets while Ken finished his paperwork. Not far ahead, I saw someone lying beneath a car. I let our dispatcher know we had come across a "ped-struck." The dispatcher asked for our exact location and then after a long pause instructed us not to respond until the police arrived. Ken and I looked at each other but shrugged our shoulders. Dispatchers were the gods in this business—we had been trained to believe that they had the big picture. If they instructed us to stay put we did exactly that. Police cars soon converged on the scene from every direction.

Ken and I waited for the police to indicate that we could move in. "Have you ever been to an accident attended by a dozen police cars before?" I asked.

"Never."

"I wonder where they found them all?"

We were waved in by an officer. "Let's go," I said.

A middle-aged male was lying prone underneath a car. Ken said, "We have a traumatic arrest here, Roz."

I advised our dispatcher by radio and got to work.

A television crew was on the scene, and I could feel the lights for their camera shining on my back. The driver of the car was hysterical. "I swear I didn't see him. He was just all of a sudden there ... I didn't see him ..."

Everything moved quickly as we attempted to resuscitate our patient. Ken said quietly, "This guy has some really weird injuries for someone who has been hit by a car. I think he's been shot."

"That would explain all the police," I answered, noting that another ambulance crew had been found to assist us. The other paramedics climbed into the back of our ambulance to try to start an intravenous while I drove the few short blocks to the hospital.

As soon as we had wheeled our patient into Emergency, I went back to the ambulance to start cleaning it out. There was blood everywhere. I looked down and noticed that my boots were covered. A crew member who was waiting for his partner came over and offered to help with the job.

"Are you guys having the same kind of night we are?" I asked. "Or are we just charmed?"

"Yeah, it's crazy," he said. "All gang-related."

"Nice city this is—"

A squeal of tires cut me off mid-sentence. A car screamed up to the Emergency entrance of the hospital. The paramedic I'd been talking to disappeared. As the car came to a sudden stop, I realized there was a second car in hot pursuit. The driver of the first car opened his door, sending particles of glass onto the pavement. He got out and I saw that his shirt was soaked in blood. Before I had a chance to move, the second car pulled up behind. Two men jumped out, revolvers clasped between their hands, arms extended straight out from the top of their doors just like in the movies. Using their doors as shields, they levelled the muzzles of their guns at the man in the first car—and at me.

I heard one of the men in the second car yell, "Freeze!" I hit the ground behind the ambulance. When I didn't hear anything more, I looked up from the road. The first driver had slumped to the ground.

I glanced at the men in the second car and decided they had to be undercover cops. I moved quickly towards the man who had collapsed. I didn't have a stretcher, but at least I had gloves. I ripped off the man's shirt and attempted to stop the bleeding. Another paramedic and a triage nurse rushed out of the hospital with a gurney.

"If this is what happens on a lunar eclipse," the nurse said, "I'll never complain about a full moon again." We pushed our way into Emergency. The medical staff looked up, surprised; no one had advised them of yet another critical patient. One of the doctors asked me for details. I explained that the patient had dropped himself off at the door; I had just happened to be there for the pick-up.

I went back to cleaning out the back of our ambulance. Finished with his patient, Ken sauntered out of the hospital. He had a big smile on his face. He made a fist and pointed his thumb back towards the Emergency entrance. "Did you just bring that last guy in?"

I grinned at him, and nodded.

"I don't believe it," he said. "Apparently the guy has been shot three times. The one we took in—the one that had been run over—had been shot twice. What is going on in this city tonight?"

"It's probably gang-related."

"No doubt. What a way to clean up the streets. We should just let them go at it." He started to laugh and I joined in. The laughter helped to reduce the tension, but I could tell we were getting punchy.

Ken gulped down a large bottle of water. I looked at my watch. It was 04:00. Our shift didn't end for a few more hours. I needed to be at the hospital shortly after that. I had thought only fleetingly of the surgery, mainly because I was so thirsty. A simple drink of water wasn't possible.

By the time we had finished cleaning the ambulance, our dispatcher advised us that the city had finally gone to sleep. He was sending us back to our station.

We were exhausted. But we knew that the adrenalin in our systems probably would keep us from getting any sleep. We stayed up and watched an old Charlie Chaplin movie, *Easy Street*, until the end of our shift.

Peter was already up and dressed when I got home. He knew at a glance what kind of night I'd had. I smiled and reminded him, "I'll get more than enough sleep soon."

Deirdre had dropped off a card with a kayaking scene on the front. Inside, she sent her love and wished me "smooth paddling."

I dropped my uniform directly into a bag for the dry cleaner, had a shower, got dressed and went downstairs to give Katherine and Jenny a big hug. I tucked Deirdre's card into my pocket, telling Peter I was ready to leave.

I closed my eyes for most of the ride to the hospital. When we arrived at Admitting, Peter asked, "Did you see the eclipse last night?"

"No." I laughed. "Believe it or not, I didn't even look."

He put his arm around my shoulders. "It was quite something," he said.

We went through the admission paperwork and then headed upstairs to day surgery. I was beginning to feel like a veteran. On went the hospital garments. And off I went to say good-bye to Peter.

"They'll call you when I'm ready to come home," I said, feeling surprisingly nonchalant.

I was wheeled into the same operating room I'd had for my mastectomy. The clock on the wall said 10:00; everything was happening right on time. I was relieved to see the same anaesthetist I'd had for my last surgery.

"You better watch how much of that stuff you give me," I warned her. "I've been working all night. I feel as if I could sleep for a week."

"I'm glad you mentioned that," she said. "It's good for me to know."

"On the other hand," I continued, "I'm still pumped up with adrenalin."

"Was it a busy night?" she asked.

"Very busy. Last night, the city was a shambles."

Dr. Harris came into the operating room. He lowered his mask and looked directly at me. "Hi, Rosalind. The lab results of the needle biopsy were inconclusive, but you're going to be just fine."

I smiled a little smile to myself but said nothing.

The anaesthetist slipped the needle into my arm, and I was out cold.

"Hello, Rosalind. Wake up. Come on now. That's the way." I knew someone was talking to me, but her voice was weirdly disembodied. I could hear my voice answering questions, but I wasn't sure what words were coming out of my mouth. I must have dozed off again, waking as I was wheeled from the recovery room back to day surgery. In the bed next to me, a woman lay motionless. A nurse took my vitals and asked me how I felt. "Nauseated," I told her. She came back with a shot of Gravol.

I woke again to hear Dr. Harris's voice. "Bad news, I'm afraid." I realized through the fog in my head that he was talking to the woman in the next bed. I heard her say something, and he responded. "The tumour is malignant."

I listened to the woman cry softly, and I felt her pain. I wondered how many times a day this man had to say those words. I waited for my turn.

Suddenly he was standing over me. I searched his face.

"The biopsy went well," he said. "I did a lumpectomy, removed an area of the breast that was about five centimetres by three centimetres by three centimetres. We did a frozen section in the operating room, and it appears that the cells were in the process of changing. We call it hyperplasia. Are you familiar with the term?"

"Yes."

"I removed a good margin of tissue around the lump, and I think that's all we'll have to do." He placed his hand lightly on my arm. "The lab results will give us the rest of the picture. Make an appointment to see me towards the end of next week."

I felt his hand give my arm a squeeze. "You can go back to sleep now," he said. And I did.

Sometime later a nurse placed a tray of tea and sandwiches in front of me. Experience told me not to touch any of it, but I was so thirsty that I gulped down the tea. Almost instantaneously, I threw it all up.

When Peter arrived to take me home, he looked at me expectantly. I realized he was waiting for information. I was so groggy I could hardly speak, but I heard myself telling him, "It looks good. The surgery looks good."

I went to bed as soon as I got home. Jenny said that Pat had dropped off a card. Jenny wanted to open it, so I told her to go ahead.

"On the front it says: 'A Mass for Your Intentions.'"

"What?" I said, lifting my head and taking the card from Jenny's hand. It was an official-looking card from a church. I read: "The Holy Sacrifice of the Mass Will Be Offered for Your Intentions—May God Keep You in His Loving Care."

I put my head back on the pillow and laughed. I couldn't stop laughing.

"What's it mean?" Jenny asked, taking the card back so she could look at it again.

"Pat has had a mass said for me."

Jenny stared at me with a blank look, uncomprehending. I tried to explain. "Well, if they've had a wake for me, why not a mass?" I was still grinning when I fell asleep.

I slept a lot over the next few days. The third anaesthetic and more blood loss within such a short period of time had taken their toll. At some point Mike, a writer friend of mine, called, and we talked for hours, bringing each other up to date. Mike used to hang around our house a lot. He was just a friend who was wild and funny and attentive—too attentive, it became apparent. One day after Mike had left, my peace-loving, anti-gun, Honda-driving husband was sitting in a chair reading a newspaper. Without looking up from his paper, he said, "Tell Mike that if he doesn't stay away from you, I'm going to throw my shotgun in the back of my pick-up and go get him."

Peter spoke lightly but without skipping a beat. His comment caught me by surprise. I laughed as I said to him, "What would I want with a man who's been married nine times?" Mike once explained that he'd asked God for nine lives, but God didn't hear him correctly and gave him nine wives. Peter had agreed that there was no harm in my keeping in touch with Mike. And we'd done exactly that.

Although I was still apprehensive about the results of the biopsy, I was in surprisingly good spirits once I'd had some rest, and I spent a ridiculous number of hours simply enjoying the world. Sometimes I wanted only to feel the sun pouring through the windows. Sometimes I'd watch an eagle coast in and out of view. Occasionally I'd do something a bit more productive. As I weeded the herbs, I appreciated the parsley that had survived another winter. Healing, I decided, was about doing anything that opened the heart.

18

PAT HAD GONE EAST to attend a family wedding. She'd left a small porcelain angel to look after me, and she called frequently. Deirdre and I had continued to talk regularly following my surgery, sometimes two or three times a day. We saw a lot of each other. She was very caring, and from that I drew a kind of strength.

Finally it was ten days after my surgery—time to have my stitches removed and to find out the results of my biopsy. Deirdre invited me to drop by for a drink afterwards. All day I made a point of concentrating on my visit with her.

I sat in the waiting room skimming through some magazines about women with perfect bodies. As a patient left one of the examination rooms I glanced up, curious. She was talking to the nurse and I could hear that she was very upset. I looked at the back of her head. She was bald. Then she turned and I saw her face. Saw the fear and despair. It made me feel ill. Despite the strange metamorphosis of losing her hair, I instantly recognized Shannon, my wardmate from the hospital. She held onto the edge of the counter as though she needed support. The nurse was unsuccessfully trying to comfort her.

I stood up, waiting for Shannon to notice me. She turned towards the door and then rushed across the waiting room blindly.

I called out, "Shannon."

She paused, met my eyes for just an instant, and then gave me a quick thumbs-down sign before continuing out the door.

Leaving my jacket on the chair, I caught up with her in the hall. There were several people waiting for the elevator.

"I can't talk," she said, breaking into a fast walk.

I put my hand on her arm and directed her gently towards a door marked "Stairway." We stood alone on a landing. Tears streamed down her face.

"It's the cancer," she sobbed. "I'm not going to make it."

I held out my arms and she fell forward into their small comfort. The moment had the tenuousness of a dream. I rocked her gently back and forth.

She whimpered, "I have to leave my babies." And then she let out a scream that took my breath away. It seemed to echo forever in the stairwell.

The exit door was pushed open, and several people stood glaring into the dimmed area, trying to see what was happening.

"It's okay, it's okay," I said to them, holding Shannon and trying to keep the door shut. She cried until it seemed she had worn herself out. I rummaged in my pocket for a tissue and waited while she blew her nose.

"Martin is waiting for me in the car," she sighed. "He's got the kids. What a mess I am."

I said softly, "When you're ready, I'll walk you down."

She closed her eyes and took another deep breath.

"Okay," she said.

I put my hand under her arm, and slowly we descended the stairs together. When we reached the outside door, she pulled a pair of sunglasses out of her pocket and put them on.

"Just stop for a minute and get some air," I suggested. I reached into my pocket for a scrap of paper and scribbled my name and phone number on it. "Shannon, please call me."

She didn't answer at first but looked at the paper and tucked it into her pocket. "What's happening with you?" she asked, staring off at a neighbouring yard full of swings and jungle gyms.

"Things are good," I heard myself say. "I'm okay."

"Thank God for that."

"Yes," I said.

We moved to let some people pass by. Although they were trying not to show it, I could sense they felt they were walking close to disaster. As I moved aside to give them room, I saw myself in Shannon's mirrored sunglasses. She gave my hand a squeeze and walked away.

I watched her cross the parking lot to a car that had children bounding about in the back seat, shrieking with laughter. Her husband was leaning against the door. When he saw Shannon approach, he walked to the middle of the parking lot and looked down at her. I could see her mouth moving. Her husband turned, put his arm around her waist. Together they walked back to their car.

When I returned to the office, one glance told me that the other patients had heard the scream. All eyes openly searched my face, and I sensed a kind of restlessness. The women had been so frightened by the magnitude of Shannon's suffering that the room had been taken over by terror. I apologized to the nurse for being away so long. She assured me that it had not been a problem and asked, "How is she?"

"She's okay now. She's with her husband."

"Oh, I'm so glad," the nurse replied. "I was worried she might be driving."

"No," I said, and sat down where I'd left my jacket.

I closed my eyes. I felt completely drained. Shannon's scream was still resounding in my head. It was almost as if it had become trapped inside me. I had heard that kind of scream before in my work. It was a sound that came from the soul. A sound full of unbearable loss. Her scream was the scream of every woman who must leave a child. It was the kind of scream that I knew I'd never ever get out of my head.

I was grateful for a few minutes to compose myself before seeing the doctor. So many times in my work I had needed to comfort people dealing with overwhelming loss. I'd often tried to find something to say, but there were no words that could lessen the grief. Touch was all that was left. I had held many people, not as a paramedic but simply as another human being. It was impossible not to feel some of their pain.

My head was still so full of Shannon's scream that I didn't hear my name being called. I opened my eyes, startled to see the nurse standing in front of me. With a concerned expression, she said, "Ms. MacPhee, the doctor can see you now—you can go right in."

As always, Dr. Harris greeted me pleasantly and asked how I was doing.

I told him, "I'm feeling lucky today."

"Wonderful," he said. I had a feeling that it wasn't a word he said a lot in this office.

"I'm feeling lucky," I explained, "because I've just talked to a woman who isn't going to make it and she has three young children at home."

He nodded his head and looked me squarely in the eyes. "But you are going to make it."

I realized I had been sitting with a kind of battered steadiness waiting for whatever he might have to say. "The pathology report showed the edges of the tissue I removed were clean," he said. "You must walk on horseshoes."

I smiled and briefly felt my body relax. He started to snip away at the black stitches.

"There," he said, stepping back to admire his work. "You have quite a hematoma, with a few rainbow colours thrown in, but it's healing nicely."

He handed me a mirror. I looked at the neat incision and said, "I figured from the amount of tissue you said you'd removed that I'd lost about a quarter of my breast. But it doesn't look any smaller."

"It's full of fluid right now. Last time you had a lumpectomy, you had your breast removed right afterwards. You didn't see what your breast would have looked like when the swelling went down."

"Well, at the moment it doesn't look so bad. Almost looks like a happy face," I said.

He smiled. "The bruising may take quite a while to clear up," he warned, washing his hands.

I was still looking at my breast from different angles in the mirror. "So when the swelling goes down, maybe my prosthesis will have to be traded in for a smaller one?"

"The breast will get smaller," he said.

"Appreciably smaller?" I asked.

"Enough to make a difference. You may see the nipple drop a little. But you still have the breast."

"Yes," I nodded. "I still have the breast."

"Do you need a prescription for something to help with the discomfort?"

"No, I still have some pills left. Compared to the other side, the pain's nothing."

"Still a lot there?" he asked.

"I'm getting used to it, but I dive into the drugs from time to time."

He made some notes in my file. "I'd like to see you again in a week just to make sure everything is healing the way we want.

And then I don't want to see you again." He smiled and added, "Unless you're dropping by to say hello."

As I drove home my thoughts drifted with all the different emotions I was feeling. Relief for myself. The possibility of hope. Such sadness for Shannon. Her cry in my head.

I called Peter, relieved to give him good news. As promised, I also called Katherine and Jenny at work. I found the number Pat had given me for her family in the east and called her too. We had a boisterous conversation.

My experience at the doctor's office had worn me out and I knew I should have a rest before going to Deirdre's, but I couldn't wait to tell her. I decided to drive over. If necessary, I'd walk home. The sun was lowering itself towards the ocean by the time I arrived at her house.

"How did it go?" she asked right away.

"Time to celebrate," I said, handing her the bottle of wine I'd brought with me. For the first time in ages, I realized I was feeling genuinely cheerful, happy. With no reservations. I grinned at her. "My doctor says I must walk on horseshoes."

"Oh, yes!" she said, slamming the bottle down on the kitchen counter. "I knew it."

"The cells were changing, but the doctor says he has cut away all the tissue that needs to be removed. No chemotherapy. No radiation."

She let out a shout and grabbed two crystal wine glasses from the cupboard. She handed me a corkscrew. "Here, you do the honours."

I noticed a single tall-stemmed rose in a glass vase strategically placed underneath a spotlight. The rose was a remarkable red. I looked down into its deep velvet richness.

I opened the wine, suddenly noticing the silence in her house. "Where is everyone?"

"Gone. They've all abandoned me for a few hours. Isn't it wonderful? It's so peaceful."

I poured two tall dark glasses of wine. We made a great show of toasting to our health and to life.

Then we sat outside. There were a few clouds directly overhead, but it was a beautiful evening. The light reflected off the distant waves. As the sun dropped into the ocean, its last light brought out the copper tones in Deirdre's hair and created interesting curves of light and shade on her face. She sat in her softness like a painting.

More and more colours appeared in the sky. The sunset turned so intensely red that it looked as if the sky were tearing away from the horizon. The air had the kind of closeness that warns of a summer storm.

Deirdre shielded her eyes. Then she said quietly, "I want to tell you something. And I don't want you to say a word. Okay?"

"Sure," I said, looking at her. She shifted in her chair.

"Remember the day you took me out to lunch?"

I nodded.

"Well, when I finally went back to my car I found I'd left my lights on. The battery was absolutely flat. So I called my hubby to pick me up." She paused and then said, "We went and looked at a house in West Vancouver. We put in an offer and it's been accepted. Isn't it crazy? All because of a dead battery, we bought a house."

The wine in my mouth felt like glass. I swallowed, willing the moment not to have happened. I clung to the interval before I had heard her words. I stared out over the ocean, then looked up at the sky. The wine in my stomach sickened me. I looked at Deirdre with blank incomprehension. What was she saying?

Her voice floated towards me. "This new place is in really rough shape … needs a pile of work … it's just down the road."

What I seemed to be stuck on was the humour she saw in buying a house many miles away "all because of a dead battery." A pain moved through me, taking my breath away. A pain that was familiar, all-pervasive; it affected every cell of my body. A voice in my head took over, issuing orders. Say nothing. Do nothing. The pain will pass. The words played over and over in my head: "All because of a dead battery, we bought a house ..."

I was surprised to hear the sound of my own voice. It was flat and strange, as if it belonged to someone else. "I'll leave you the wine," I said. And I fled, leaving her to it.

I opened the car door and slid into the driver's seat. I sat there, stunned. The sky, so cruelly hacked and gouged, had striations of black running through it. Although I'd only had a few sips of wine, I felt drunk. I nursed the car home slowly. I seemed to be floating with Shannon's scream locked inside. I pulled into my driveway, turned the ignition off and leaned forward against the steering wheel. I cried so violently my body shook. I was aware I'd stopped only when I heard raindrops splattering on the windshield. Both sides of my face were soaked in warm tears.

Grateful that no one was home, I made my way inside and put my head down on the dining room table. I closed my eyes and stayed like that for a long time. I had the sensation of my head being held under water. The words of the young Mexican drifted through my head: "Never turn your back to the ocean." I had turned my back, and now a big one, a sleeper, had taken me down.

I sat by the window until the darkness set in and there was nothing left to see. I carried a book over to the sofa and lay down. I heard a lightning crack to the east, but when I looked out the window there was only an empty space before the darkness closed in again. The words on the page swam. I listened as a sudden gust of wind slammed branches against the roof and walls. The lamp by my head blinked intermittently. I fell asleep, then awakened, then fell asleep again—always to the howl of the storm. At some point in the night, someone placed a quilt over me and turned off the light.

I felt very ill in the morning. I opened my eyes to see Peter bustling about, packing a suitcase. He apologized for being so late getting home but said he'd had to prepare a brief for his business trip. We talked about my doctor's appointment, and then about the storm. The sky was now so blue it was as if we'd imagined the wild weather of the night before.

"Do you know how long you'll be away?" I asked him.

"Probably until the end of the week. I'll phone," he said, walking over to the sofa. He bent down and gave me a kiss. "You fell asleep reading last night."

"I seem to have come down with a cold," I sniffled.

"Take more time off. Get someone to cover your shifts."

"But I want to get back to work. It's good for me in other ways. Where are the kids?"

"Jenny stayed at Jen's place. Katherine's asleep downstairs." He gave me a good-bye kiss. "Love you," he said.

"Love you," I said, watching him back out the door with his suitcase. For a long time I did nothing but watch the early light climb the far wall. Then I got up slowly and sat at the edge of the sofa. I was in pain. *Battery … battery … all because of a dead battery.* Little words. Nothing words.

A single swift blow had left me so weak I could hardly move. Emotions I felt I shouldn't have flooded me. Fear. Aloneness. Profound disappointment. But most of all, anger. Deirdre had bailed out because of my cancer, I thought. I wanted to use whatever time I had in this world to focus on people I loved.

She wanted to focus on a new house. Did she think friendships like ours were commonplace? We had seen each other through all manner of ups and downs, celebration, illness, injury and death. Had I expected too much to think that would continue? I couldn't make sense out of any of it.

I was filled with defeat, a defeat so deep and unconditional that the sense of reality had been sucked out of everything around me. I wanted to scream, "Enough, I've had enough." But instead, I buried myself in Deirdre's words until I felt nothing but their weight. Perhaps if I had stayed to talk with her. But she had asked me not to say anything. And I'd been paralyzed by an intensity of feeling that overwhelmed whatever I might have said. I had walked away because I didn't want her to know I needed her. I had walked away because I knew if I stayed, I'd blow my whole act of bravado. And my act was all I had left.

As one week passed into the next, I did whatever was expected of me, but I felt disconnected from everything, almost as if I were watching someone else play me in a movie. I acquired the ability to freeze-frame each thought. Cut. Fade. Fast-forward to the next. Replay over and over.

I didn't say a word to my family about Deirdre's pending move. It seemed to me there was no point in telling them. What good would it have done? Besides, I didn't feel capable of telling them. They suspected nothing beyond my suffering of a stubborn cold along with post-surgical fatigue. Although I knew I was putting on the performance of my life, I was relieved, and amazed, that everyone was oblivious to what was happening inside me. Or so I thought.

At lunch one day, Katherine sat across from me at the table. She leaned forward, resting her chin in her hands, regarding me as I chewed away at a chicken bone.

"I'm amazed you still eat that stuff," she said stiffly.

"I have vastly improved," I assured her. "This is free-range stuff, organic stuff—it's stuff that saw blue sky."

"Knowing how you feel about blue sky, I can see how that would be important to you."

"No, really," I said in self-defence. "I'm into vegetables and grains, I've cut way back on my fats, I drink skim milk with my Kahlúa now, I eat hardly any refined or processed foods any more—"

"Okay, okay," she said, cutting me off with a grin.

I waved the chicken bone at her threateningly. "Let me tell you something else—the only reason we can eat this *stuff* is because we have two incomes in this family. Without money, we'd be eating meat treated with hormones and food full of chemicals."

She pondered this quietly and sat watching me eat. Then, out of the blue, she said, "I saw a For Sale sign at Deirdre's."

"Yep," I answered, looking away. I felt her eyes search my face.

"Where are they going?"

"West Vancouver," I said as casually as I could.

"Oh, that's not so bad," she said, pausing before she added, "I guess."

"No," I agreed. I changed the topic abruptly. "How's the studying of anaphylaxis and angioneurotic edema doing?" We settled comfortably into shoptalk. She was sensitive enough not to push the subject.

I continued to pretend that Deirdre's move was the most inconsequential thing in the world. But a numbness stayed with me. I went to work, walked the dog, did the shopping. I believed I was doing a competent job at everything. But I felt so sad and battle-weary that I was hardly recognizable to myself.

My needs didn't jibe with her needs, I reasoned. I couldn't understand it in any other way. I thought it was strange that I might have had cancer for more than eight years and that everything had hummed along, more or less fine, during that time. It was only with the diagnosis and treatment that everything had turned upside-down.

I'd never been good at handling separations or good-byes. I suspected that a long history of losing people I loved, starting at a very young age, had something to do with it. This time the grief and anger were overpowering. I remembered hearing of a woman who had an excellent reputation as a grief counsellor. Maybe, I said to myself. Maybe—

Just after I'd made an appointment to see the counsellor, I answered the phone and heard Pat's cheerful voice. "And how are *we* today?"

"Welcome home," I said. "I've missed you, missed you."

"And I have missed you," she answered. "But you sound dreadful. You sound like you need some homemade chicken soup with rice."

"It's just a cold," I said, then corrected myself. "Actually, two colds, I think. One coming and one going—"

"Listen," she interrupted. "Are you up and about?"

"Yes, but I'm not terribly good company."

"Not to worry. Let's get together."

I knew she'd see through me. "I can't, Pat. Don't take it personally. I just don't want to share my cold with you."

"Rosalind, I need to talk to you—your place or mine?"

I hesitated for a moment. "I could drop by ... in a bit."

"Perfect. I'll start the soup right now."

A basket of flowers propped her front door open. I called out to her as I walked in.

"Soup's on," she said from the kitchen. Despite my cold, I could smell its wonderful aroma.

She gave me a hearty embrace and then stepped back to say, "You look awful."

"Thanks a lot." I smiled at her. Her face had an exuberant colour. "*You* look great."

Her eyes darted across my face. She linked her arm through mine and drew me out onto the deck. She whispered, "Let's you and I have a little drink," as if we were in a room full of people and she didn't want anyone to hear.

We stood side by side at the railing, sipping our drinks and taking in the view of ocean and mountains. She told me a few amusing stories about her visit in the east. Finally she said, "I don't know how to say this, so I'm just going to come out with it. I've heard a little rumour. I've heard that Deirdre has her house on the market."

I nodded.

"Rosalind, how are you handling that?"

I had to swallow before I could answer. "Not well."

She let out a deep sigh. "Oh, I don't like you being hurt." She put her arm lightly on my shoulder. "Have you any idea why they are moving?"

I shook my head.

"Are you as shocked as I am? I mean, they already have such a magnificent house. Have they sold their place yet?"

"I don't know."

"You don't really want to talk about this, do you?" she said.

I made a bit of smile, grateful, and didn't try to explain.

"Then just let me say something. This may or may not apply to you—that's for you to decide. I seem to be forever going back to when the boys were killed, but so often I've seen a disaster happen in someone's life and then everything else seems to go ass-over-tea-kettle at the same time. As you know, I had some interesting friendship challenges right after the boys died."

I nodded.

"Well, after the slide, our whole family went to a shrink, not because we couldn't handle what had happened so much as I just felt the family should receive counselling. There was such potential for future difficulties. The shrink was a wonderful woman, and one of the things she said has remained with me: 'Someone can't be what you want them to be—they just are what they are.'"

"I don't think Deirdre is into the breast cancer scene," I said shakily. "She told me herself that she didn't need this in her life right now."

"Well, if that's the case, I think her move is quite ingenious ... but it's her loss. I'm *into* things like death and dying."

I choked on my drink, but I actually laughed. "What do you mean?"

She smiled, but there was a discernible seriousness to her voice. "Well, death is kind of seductive. It's dramatic, it's exciting, it cuts through all the shit. Roz, it's supposed to bring people closer together."

"Not always, Pat, not always." I smiled and shook my head. "If anyone knows, you must—we live with our losses."

"Oh, I don't like this," she complained. With a dismissive wave of the hand, she said, "Let's have some chicken soup."

She held the door open for me and I followed her back inside. "Feast," she said, putting a bowl in front of me.

We ate quietly for a moment or two, but I could see she was still mulling over Deirdre's move. Finally she asked, "Roz, am I imagining it, or have you and Deirdre been out of sync for a while?"

I studied my bowl of soup. "Cancer has made everything different. Deirdre seems no longer herself; maybe *I'm* no longer *myself*."

"People change," she said thoughtfully. "With every experience we become slightly different people. We think the people we love are changing with us. But often, this is not the case."

"Well, I guess Deirdre has things happening in her life that are changing her too." I put my spoon down, stared at the bottom of my bowl as if I could see something there, and said, "I'm really going to miss her."

Pat kept her eyes on me. "You know something, Roz?" she asked, without waiting for an answer. "Deirdre hasn't been where you have been ... and she isn't where you are now."

"I know." I sighed. "I've been muddling along the best I can. It's just that—" I cut myself off.

"You're really having difficulty with this, aren't you?"

"Well, I'm walking, talking ... drinking. I just feel so numb."

"Does talking about it help or make it worse?"

"Actually, I've made an appointment to see a grief counsellor next week."

"Good for you."

I tried to smile. "Well, I figure you're nothing nowadays unless you're grieving, mourning or healing—so why not?"

She laughed. "I'm proud of you."

I pushed myself away from the table, making ready to leave. I kissed her lightly on her cheek. "Thank you, my friend," I said. "As always, a thousand thank yous."

"Will you be okay?" she asked.

I looked at her.

"Okay getting home?"

"I'll be okay."

She gave a regal wave of her hand as I drove off.

19

THE DAY I WAS TO see the counsellor, I wandered the house vacantly for a long while. Finally I showered and dressed. I opened the deck doors for some fresh air, watched a squirrel, made coffee in the kitchen and lingered over a piece of toast. When I couldn't think of any other ways to delay my departure, I nudged myself out the door. Lots of people nowadays seemed to think nothing of running off to a therapist with their problems, but I found it to be a significant step. I couldn't imagine revealing my hidden self to a stranger. Yet in my own efforts to work through all that had happened, there had been no revelations, only a huge sadness.

The counsellor's office was empty except for carpet and two chairs. She was a woman about my age. After I finished explaining why I had come to her, we sat silently. Still. Waiting, it seemed. It was pleasantly Zen.

"One of the hardest things we learn in life is that we can have no control over the actions of other people." She said this slowly, carefully. I brought my hands together on my lap and stared at them, giving her words weight in my head. I heard her voice continue. "From what you've said, it sounds like you lost the luxury of being a child at a very early age. Your parents broke a trust." She waited another moment before she said, "There would have been a sense of abandonment as a child, and that may be what you're feeling now."

I thought this over, annoyed that a few tears had made their way to my eyes. When she asked me to tell her more about my childhood, I shifted my gaze from my hands to the high windows, and then back to her. Taking a deep breath to compose myself, I picked over the words in my mind. I heard myself say, "It's too complicated a story to tell."

I thought that would be enough, but I could see from her face that she wanted more. I smiled, just barely, and shook my head no.

"You've had a lot of things happen to you that you've had no control over," she reminded me. "You must remember that you didn't create these situations—you responded to them."

I took a slow breath. "I know everybody carries around a jumble of senseless ideas in their heads—it's just that I normally see myself as handling everything well."

Her expression was one of pleasant concern. "You can't get through life helping others and pretending you're never one of the needy."

I nodded, feeling we were back on safer ground. "It's interesting," I said. "So many people have told me how wonderfully well I'm doing. I mean, that's important to hear. But sometimes it has been enough to make me want to scream. I may have seemed stoic and reasonable and accommodating." I laughed briefly. "I may even have seemed fucking perfect at times. But I don't think anyone goes through this experience doing 'wonderfully well.' "

She smiled. We talked about how anyone who loses a part of his or her body goes into mourning. How a woman who has had a mastectomy is also mourning the destruction of her body image. The counsellor called it symbolic castration. She peered thoughtfully at me for a moment, and then said, "Your relationship with both your body and your life has changed—now your relationship with a friend has changed."

I shifted in my seat. *All because of a battery* … little words, nothing words. "Of course," I said, "I know another person is never the solution. It's just that … I should be concentrating on dealing with cancer right now, not a problem with friendship."

We sat without speaking for a few moments. I glanced at the closed door. I knew a receptionist was hard at work on the other side, and there were other counsellors in nearby offices, but the room was so quiet that I felt we were the only people in the building.

"It's really quite embarrassing," I said suddenly. "I mean, I feel my reaction is absurd. A friend has been out looking at houses without telling me. So what?"

She nodded. "You're forgetting that your reaction comes at a time when you have enormous needs of your own. What many cancer patients discover is that they can no longer ignore their own needs."

I closed my eyes, going back to the moment when Deirdre had told me she and her husband had bought a new house. "It was just such a shock," I said. "The way she told me. Maybe it wouldn't have made any difference, but I wish she'd given me some warning. She loved her home. That she might move was as unlikely as my getting cancer." I listened to my words settle in the silence.

"Betrayal is wherever it is perceived," she said finally. "It may be betrayal by a person or betrayal by a body. You've been dealing with both."

I tossed my head back as if I needed to shake something off. "I'm sure she wouldn't look at it that way. She probably thinks I'm a lousy friend if I can't care about her the same way regardless of where she lives. But I know we won't end up seeing much of each other, and I guess— I guess I'd naively thought we were in each other's survival plan."

"How would you have liked her to tell you she was moving?"

"I suppose ... if she'd sounded like she cared and maybe said, 'Listen, you and I have to work around something that has come up.' Or, 'We have come across our dream home and an opportunity of a lifetime that we just can't pass up.' Something that made some sense." I checked myself from saying anything more.

The woman stood up and walked around behind me. "When your friend told you she was moving, what reaction would you have expected from yourself?"

I stared at the empty chair. "To be happy for her because she was doing what she wanted to do. I would like to have said: 'How exciting—let me help you pack.'"

"Let me reword my question—how would you have expected someone else to react if she were in your shoes?"

"I wouldn't have expected so much, I guess." I hesitated. "It's hard to explain, but suddenly a clock presides over everything I do. For me, the time for our friendship is *now*. She wants to put her *now* time into a house."

The counsellor slipped back into her chair. She said, "Most people think of death as being the ultimate separation. I've always felt that to lose someone you love who chooses to be elsewhere is the ultimate challenge."

"To her, it's just moving down the road."

"Twenty miles away is not 'just down the road.' You know that, but perhaps she doesn't." She studied me for a moment or two, and then said, "You know, it's possible that your friend may not be aware of your needs right now."

I flattened myself against the firmly cushioned chair. "Can she simply not know her closest friend has been hit by lightning?"

"She may have chosen not to know, or *she* may not be able to deal with this right now. You said she's been in mourning herself. Denial may be part of her survival."

If she had been planning to say more, I preempted her. "I know it's not rational, but on an emotional level I feel she wouldn't have moved if I didn't have cancer," I said. I caught myself thinking of Deirdre as a teen-ager, losing her mother to breast cancer. I swallowed before I added, "I even feel *guilty* for having cancer."

With the calm assurance of someone who had said the words countless times before, she replied, "Feelings are inside us all, working on us, no matter how we deal with things on any other level." She leaned forward in her chair. "You must remember that you are still in enormous emotional shock from the diagnosis. It can take a person years to adjust to having cancer." She paused. "Tell me, how do you feel you've managed the loss of the breast? A lot of women have trouble with that."

I felt a strange trembling deep inside myself. I ran one of my hands through my hair. "That's been much harder than I ever thought it would be—the unattractiveness of it all. A day doesn't go by when I don't look down and gasp at the shock of my missing breast. I simply can't believe it's not there. It's like not knowing my own body. I know it sounds ridiculous—"

"It's a normal reaction," she said. "I've talked to women who can't look in a mirror for years afterwards. Do you feel you are working that out?"

"Oh, yes. I mean, as far as I'm concerned, it was the breast or my life. It's strange—neither of my doctors ever asked me about my sex life. If they had, I'd probably have told them that my husband didn't write me off, but I wrote myself off."

I could hear a siren approaching in the distance. I glanced at the blue sky beyond the window. "I think it's something doctors *should* ask. I think it's something every woman may need help with."

She nodded. "What you said about feeling guilt—a lot of women feel that way. It's also not uncommon for a woman to feel ashamed of her body after a mastectomy."

"Yes, I can see that. There are daily reminders when bathing, dressing ... making love. It must be very difficult for women on their own. I've had tremendous support from my husband, daughters and friends. That's made an incredible difference."

"You're lucky."

I raised my voice over the sound of the siren. "Yes. Ironically, I'm learning that more and more since I've had cancer—how lucky I am."

We listened together as the siren passed by.

"Ambulance?" she asked.

I nodded and smiled, looking at my watch.

"One more question, if I may. What are you going to do about your friend?"

"I'll call her. I've been feeling that she's the one who should make the effort, offer some kind of explanation, but who knows." I stood up, getting ready to leave. "Anyway, she hasn't ... so I'll call. And then I'll just get on with it."

"Good for you," she said, walking me to the door. She put her hand on my shoulder in a gesture of support. "My suggestion is that you determine your priorities. Make a list of what you'd expect from someone else who has been through what you've been through and work from there. I wish you luck."

I drove home deep in thought, mulling over everything we'd discussed. I kept going back to various events in my childhood. I wondered if parents could really create so much trouble even though they were gone.

I had many early memories of love, but many of fear as well. First, I had been afraid for myself. Then for my parents. My ten-year-old self had known on some level that my father would take his life. My bones told me. My blood told me. When he jumped to his death, I believed I had allowed it to happen.

I was only now beginning to understand that the loss of my mother to depression had been equally devastating. Withdrawn was not dead. But, like my father, she had chosen to be somewhere else. She suffered terribly from some kind of condition, possibly agoraphobia. I nursed her for years. My two oldest sisters had already married, and the next two were soon gone. They stayed away, I supposed, for their own survival. I didn't know for sure. It had never seemed important before. We had been brought up to keep our troubles to ourselves.

The landscape passed as a blur. I checked the speedometer and eased my foot off the gas, slipping into fifth gear.

Although my mother hadn't been able to take on the role of care-giver, she had given me something very important. In every way she could, she let me know it wasn't *me* that was wrong, but the situation I was in. A teacher and a neighbouring family reinforced that. When I was a teen-ager and life started to seem like too much trouble, neighbours took me into their home. What a difference all those people made to my life. They gave me safe places to go. They praised and encouraged me. They allowed me to believe that I was good at things and that I had something to offer. Without saying it, they made me feel I could withstand terrible storms. They also gave me an unmistakable sense of community.

I pulled out to the left and overtook a semi hauling a heavy load. In my rearview mirror, I saw it grow smaller and smaller.

Strange that I'd never really talked about my parents to anyone. One reason, I suspected, was loyalty. After all, they had made me feel loved and lovable. I remembered them as extraordinary people who had screwed up. I'd always felt that they'd done their best. But there was still a lot I didn't understand. There were many black holes in the memories of my childhood. Deirdre had once suggested that if my parents were around to tell their stories, I might find it easier to tell my own.

People can only act out of their life experiences, the counsellor had said. A line from *Hiroshima, Mon Amour* came back to me: *A living creature is a memory that acts.* That concept applied to Deirdre's life too, I realized.

As I pulled into our driveway, I was glad I'd seen the counsellor. I felt as though I'd been to church. Perhaps it was an act of faith, I thought, just to believe that problems were solvable.

I waited for a day when I wasn't working and had the house to myself. It was exactly a month since I had last seen Deirdre. I thought it strange that we had not come face to face in the street or anywhere else since then.

It was almost noon when I called. She answered right away.

"Deirdre, would you have time to come over and talk?"

There was a long pause, and then she said, "Yes, if you do." Her tone was hard and dismissive.

"Are you busy now?"

"In a half hour?"

"Fine."

"See you then."

While I waited for her, I made some coffee. We had all been wounded, I thought, and we all had the power to help someone heal. A good friendship was about being able to switch those positions back and forth. I wondered what had happened to us.

When she arrived, we gave each other a cautious and cool embrace. Her face showed nothing.

"Coffee?" I asked.

"Sure," she said, removing her jacket and draping it over the back of the chair.

I filled two cups and carried them to the table. I struggled to think of the right thing to say and inhaled to compose myself. "I felt you and I have shared enough history that we should talk."

She nodded, saying nothing.

"When you told me you were moving I walked away because I couldn't handle one thing more."

She studied her coffee mug for a moment and then spoke in almost a whisper. "I know I didn't tell you the right way."

"I was in shock. I couldn't believe what I was hearing— there had been no warning."

She looked at me piercingly for a moment, then said, "There had been no warning because there had been no planning."

"You honestly just bought a house out of the blue? You know, most people *sleep* on decisions like that."

"Just a sec here. You seem to have forgotten we've never stayed in one place as long as we've stayed in Lions Bay. I have a husband who likes looking at houses. He saw this one. Someone else had just made an offer. We either had to buy it or pass it up." She kept staring at her coffee mug. "Maybe it was fate ... or maybe it was just a dead battery."

"Please don't call it fate. And don't bring the dead battery into this. If you need to call it something, call it chance, or coincidence, or *choice*—your favourite word."

She smiled slightly, more with her eyes than with her mouth. "Listen, I know I didn't tell you the right way."

"You were incredibly flip."

"You should know me well enough to know that's the way I get when I'm talking about something that really matters to me."

I had to swallow before I could continue. "You treated it as a lark. I couldn't have been more surprised—"

"Imagine my surprise," she broke in, "at finding out that our friendship depended on my address."

"It makes a huge difference. Now every time we see each other we'll have to plan it. None of this impromptu getting together—none of the drinking and walking home."

"I realize that now," she said softly, "but I didn't realize it then."

I looked at her, but she still seemed to be concentrating on her coffee mug. I decided to let her comment slide. I'd let her work that one out for herself.

"I'm sorry," she said.

We both sat silently, holding our mugs. Neither one of us had taken a sip.

"Want me to heat up your coffee?" I asked.

"No, thanks," she replied. "You know, it's ironic that I wouldn't allow the For Sale sign to go up, or anyone in the family to tell *anyone*, until I had told you, for fear that you would be upset if you heard from someone else."

"Of course I would have been upset. If I'd gone out and bought a house and you'd heard about it from someone else, wouldn't you have been upset?"

"I suppose so."

"I mean, have I just imagined the kind of friendship we've had all these years?"

"No, you haven't. I didn't want to say anything to you until you'd received the results of the biopsy. I was so happy to hear the results were good that something like a change in my address didn't seem that important."

"Deirdre, my results were better than they might have been. But I was still in shock. It wasn't just a biopsy—I had about a quarter of my remaining breast removed. Changing cells are changing cells. Regardless of how I may have seemed to you, I was pretty shaky just then."

I felt my eyes moisten a little, so I put my glasses on the table. I glanced at her and saw a frightening fierceness, but I couldn't resist a different tactic. "I was making every effort to be bright and cheery because I felt if you saw signs that I might croak of breast cancer, you'd take off."

She looked deep in thought, and then said, "Things have changed between us. I don't know, maybe it is the cancer."

I glanced out the window and saw nothing. Despite Deirdre's history of seeing things the way she wanted them to be, she had an honesty that often startled me.

"You know, I've had some pretty dark moments through all of this myself," she said slowly, choosing her words. "I've been in mourning for my father, sorting through things that contain a lot of memories—I feel I've been in a holding pattern since he died. And then everything around me started to go wrong. I was emotionally wasted. I didn't have anything left to give."

I could hear the clicking of the ceiling fan. Finally I responded. "I guess it was just lousy timing for us both."

She nodded but remained silent.

"Listen," I said. "I just want us to be able to give each other a hug and get on with our lives. I couldn't imagine bumping into you somewhere and not feeling good about seeing you."

She placed her hand lightly on mine and looked me straight in the face the way she always did when she wanted something to sink in. "Rosalind, there won't be any difference when I move. I promise you. I will see that there won't be any difference."

I smiled in uncertain relief.

She rummaged in the pocket of her jacket, pulling out a page that had been torn neatly from a magazine. She handed me my glasses, saying with a grin, "Here, put these back on so you can think intelligently again."

She carefully unfolded the page. "There ... I wanted to show you this."

She stood behind me, her hand on my shoulder, and we both looked down at the picture. It was a photo of a nude woman with one breast. The woman's face was tilted upwards towards the light and her arms were outstretched towards the sky as though to hold the sun. The scar where her breast had been was tattooed with the image of a tree branch. There was a bird in the branch.

Deirdre said, "She has a gorgeous body, don't you think?"

I nodded and picked up the page. I started to read the words written below the picture. The woman's name was Deena Metzger. She was described as a writer, lecturer and activist who lived in California. I couldn't take my eyes off her. I thought, Now that looks sexy. It gave me hope.

"May I keep the picture?"

"I brought it for you."

I stood up, holding the page with both hands. Deirdre continued, "You know, sometimes people just go along doing the best they can ... and everything seems to go wrong. I figure all a person can do is learn something from the experience and try to do better in the future. Do you agree?" she asked.

I nodded vaguely.

"Well, I can see the picture has your full attention." She was laughing now.

"Yes," I agreed. "It's full of—" I paused, looking for the right word "—possibilities."

"It's loaded with sexual power, is what it is," she said, shoving her chair back in place.

I put the picture down on the table. "I'll go with you to the car," I offered.

"Actually, I walked over."

"Then I'll walk you to the door."

We gave each other a hug that had a bit of the old warmth in it. I waved her off. It seemed we had both managed to inflict a deep hurt where none had been intended—almost as if, for a time, we had become strangers to one another. I closed the door, feeling the stillness that she had left behind. I went back upstairs, picked up the picture of the woman with the tattoo and took it to my desk. I placed the picture beside another clipping I had come across in my research. It was a photograph of a sculpture by a mastectomy patient named Nancy Fried. Her one-breasted headless torso made a significant statement to me: *The art of seeing must be learned.* I pinned the two pictures to the wall of my study.

I worked at getting my life back to some kind of normality. I kept up my exercise program and my physiotherapy. I continued to do research and even attended some meetings organized by women with breast cancer.

I dragged my friend Donna to one of the meetings. A panel of experts sat on a stage and responded to a barrage of questions from a theatre full of women with breast cancer.

As we were leaving, Donna said, "You know, every time I get a pain, I still think: Oh boy, this is it."

"Donna, I'm surprised. It's been over five years for you."

"I know, I know—it's all quite incomprehensible, isn't it?"

We both started to laugh.

I heard a woman's voice say, "Hello there. Do you remember me?"

I looked in the direction of the voice. "It's Jacki from Montreal!"

"Listen," she said, "I've moved out here now. I'm assuming we have all attended this meeting for the same reason—"

Donna grinned. "It's kind of like belonging to an exclusive club, isn't it?"

"It is, and what a wonderful club with such amazing women. It's just unfortunate the cost of membership is so dear. But listen, could we get together one day—at a civilized hour— for lunch?"

We exchanged phone numbers as we moved towards the theatre exit. Jacki asked, "What do you think about all this talk suggesting that breast cancer is linked to loss and stress? I mean, from what one doctor was saying tonight, you'd think cancer started in the heart."

"I know. It's frightening, isn't it?" Donna said. She turned to me. "Roz, you've had your nose in the books. What do you think?"

"I think that stress can negatively affect anyone's immune system, but that's as far as I'm willing to take the concept. It seems more likely to me that breast cancer is a disease with multiple causes. And if that's the case, we'd better hope they find a cure or some kind of immunotherapy."

"Like they did for polio or smallpox," Donna said.

I nodded. "There's too much emphasis placed on stress nowadays—it seems to have been in fashion, gone out of fashion, and then come back again. Dr. Susan Love thinks it's a load of rubbish. I personally think it's more like grapes."

"Grapes?" they said at the same time.

"Yes. Pliny, a Roman writer, said that the painter Zeuxis had painted some grapes in such a perfect way that birds would come by and peck at them."

Donna laughed. "Come on, Roz, there's got to be a punch line."

"Well, it's an example of an invented truth, something being so lifelike or believable that it is taken to be the real thing."

Jacki laughed. "She makes more sense at five in the morning."

"What it means," I continued, "is that the stress picture is being presented so attractively we're ready to go for it."

"Like a decoy," Donna suggested.

"Well," Jacki said, "one thing is sure: we have to get the word out, because people have got to know the numbers that go along with this disease. And *women*," she said, "have got to stop thinking that if they avoid learning about the disease, they'll avoid the disease itself."

"The art of seeing must be learned," I said.

"I think this poor girl has been in the sun too much," Jacki laughed, as we said good-bye in the darkness of the street. I stood there for a long time, looking up at the stars crowding the immense night sky.

20

THE TELEPHONE WOKE ME EARLY. It was Elaine, calling from thirty thousand feet over Greenland, words travelling to a satellite and then back to earth. As soon as I heard her voice, I glanced at the Picasso postcard beside my bed. She said she was on her way home from Paris but was leaving for China in a day or two.

"China?"

"Yes, isn't it wonderful? I've been invited to work in a hospital in Beijing for three weeks."

"I'm delighted for you," I said. "I knew you'd soon be off to some other place, but I was hoping we might see each other briefly before you left."

"I know," she said, sounding disappointed. "I do want to see you, but this came up unexpectedly and it's a great opportunity. Listen, you've been so much in my thoughts. And then last night, I dreamed about you. Are you okay?"

I was still sleepy and I had been caught off guard. Despite the miles between us, I decided to tell her. She listened quietly, asking me a few questions from time to time about the treatments I'd received.

Finally I said, "When you get back, my biochemist-turned-herbalist friend, I'm going to become your patient. I have so much to learn."

"I tell you, Roz, we have got to get back to organic farming or we are all lost."

"From everything I've read, I tend to agree with you."

"How have you been coping with all the stress of this?" she asked.

I let out a strange little laugh. "I've been better."

"Sounds like you could use a little herbal help. Get yourself some Vitamin C, Vitamin E and beta-carotene. They're good for supporting the immune system and they're also antioxidants."

"I've been taking Vitamins C and A," I informed her.

"How much?"

"A gram of Vitamin C a day and ten thousand units of Vitamin A."

"That's a good start, but you'll probably need more. I usually recommend taking Vitamin A as beta-carotene, because the body gets rid of excess beta-carotene. If you take too much Vitamin A, it accumulates in the liver."

"How about selenium? I've read that women with breast cancer tend to be low in it."

"That's true," she said. "But watch how much you take. A little is good. Too much is bad. Don't take any more than a hundred milligrams a day."

We talked for several more minutes. She said she'd put together a list of supplements and foods to add to my diet, and a list of things to take out of my diet, too. She told me to eat only wild fish and organic meat. "And go easy on the dairy products, Roz."

I laughed. "Thanks for the advice, Elaine. But you didn't call me at international rates to talk nutrition."

"Oh, but I did. Listen, I'll be back in less than a month. We'll get together. There are all kinds of things I'd like to suggest—meditation, massage, old-fashioned relaxation."

"I think I might be able to live that long."

"You'd better," she shouted with exaggerated outrage.

There was a strange buzz on the line. "Elaine, before I lose you, how was your time in Paris?"

"Paris was wonderful," she said. "I have so much to tell you. When I get back."

"Hey, thanks for calling—it has been great just to hear your voice. And good luck in China."

"Oh, Roz …"

"Yes?"

"Something to keep in mind: when Picasso painted a breast, the other one did not exist for him."

"Thanks." I laughed. "You should see the one that's left. It could use a little art."

"Bye," she called softly, and the connection was gone.

Day by day, week by week, I started making decisions. I applied to the University of British Columbia, and was accepted, as a Masters student in Fine Arts. I thought taking the writing program might buy me some time to work on manuscripts that had been collecting dust at home. I changed the title of a poetry manuscript I had started before my cancer was diagnosed: *The Forever Sky* became *Thanks for the Blue Morning*.

I bought myself a jeep because I had always wanted one. I could never have rationalized this indulgence before I had breast cancer, but I could now. A jeep would keep me close to the mountains.

I took possession of the jeep a few days before Donna's party. Donna had announced recently that she and her new husband were moving to Port Moody—an hour's drive from Lions Bay.

"Donna," I complained, "that's so far away, it might as well be Africa."

"I'll have a luncheon," she promised. "That'll get you out there."

The party had a safari theme, so I decided to dress for the occasion. I went to my friend Carol's costume store and rented a gorilla outfit. Carol sewed a pink bow to the big furry head.

I had Jenny, who never wanted to be out of my shiny new jeep, drive me to the party. A few blocks from Donna's house, I asked her to pull over. By the side of the road, she helped me climb into my costume. "Well," I said, "how do I look?"

She burst into laughter. "I don't know what you're saying—I can't hear you through that thing."

"It's so hot in here I could die," I shouted, heaving myself back into the jeep. Jouncing along, I waved at passing motorists, who honked their horns and waved in return.

When we got close to Donna's, I grabbed my bouquet of flowers and lumbered across her neighbour's lawn. I waited for Jenny to drive off, then knocked on the front door. Grunting, I presented Donna with the flowers when she answered. She hooted with laughter. Encouraged, I swaggered into the house, peering curiously at each person, inclining my head this way and that.

"Who on earth is it?" someone asked, managing to stop laughing for a moment.

I heard Pat say, "Beats me," before she cracked up again. She reached into a basket and offered me a banana.

"I need a drink," I roared, spotting a number of bottles in her basket.

"What's she saying?" two voices chimed in. "Who is it, anyway?"

I stood before a full-length mirror, shrugging my shoulders, scratching my head as if I couldn't figure out who I was. Then I caught sight of Deirdre. I loped across the carpet, dragging my arms. She stepped back, laughing. I threw a long arm around her shoulders and looked out at everyone. These were the people who had seen me through one of the wildest adventures of my life. These were my friends. I waved and did a quick little two-step.

"It's gotta be Roz," several of them shouted at the same time. I jumped up and down, nodding my head.

"Squeeze in, everybody." Pat's voice rose above the rest. Inside the huge head, I smiled. The shutter clicked. Another grouping, another pose, another click.

On the sly, I started reading about tattoos. They had been around for thousands of years and historically were presumed to have powers to protect and heal. I decided I wanted one. One of Picasso's erotically charged female figures would do just fine. I zipped my prosthesis into its little carrying case and said a fond farewell to it. I decided that if a man liked Picasso's art, he'd like my body. But I missed my breast. And although Peter never complained, I knew he missed it too.

Shannon never did call me. But she turned up in my life again. Brian and I had been sent to transfer a patient from palliative care to the Cancer Agency. When I looked at the name on the hospital chart I knew who it had to be. Turning the pages of her medical records, I was shocked that her cancer had advanced so quickly.

When I arrived in Shannon's room, she was sitting up, eating. She didn't seem at all surprised to see me. She'd lost a lot of weight since I'd seen her last. A little bit of her hair had grown back in. She was on a morphine IV pump, which meant that whenever she needed pain relief she just had to push a button. She asked me to stand on her left side since she had a problem with her vision if she looked towards the right.

I glanced around her room. There were lots of flowers. There were coloured photos of a happy smiling family. There was another picture on the wall opposite the foot of her bed; her home, I guessed. A number of toys and children's books were strewn about.

Her lunch, which was mostly liquid, sat barely touched on a tray. She was eating Jell-O, all she was able to keep down these days, she said. I could tell by the movement of her arm that she was losing her coordination. As she brought the spoon up to her mouth, the Jell-O fell onto the bed. A strange little sound came out of her mouth. She pushed the tray away and said, "I don't know why I bother."

I explained that we had come to take her to the Cancer Agency for assessment by a doctor. Brian and I helped her stand up. Brian remained in front to support her, teasing that they were dancing, while I slipped the ambulance stretcher sideways underneath her.

Once we were on our way, she gave me a perplexed, annoyed look. "So, what have you done to eradicate breast cancer since you got out of hospital?" she demanded.

"Well, I've started a book," I told her.

She looked skeptical, and I could see that this was not what she had in mind. "A book?"

"Yes," I said, wrapping the blood pressure cuff around her arm.

"Are you a writer?"

"Yes. And I've recently studied film," I said, pausing as I took the blood pressure reading. "In film they say nothing exists unless you show it. That's what I'm going to do. I'm going to show it." I wrote the numbers for her vitals on an ambulance form.

"Good. Maybe I can relax a little. I've been lying in that crummy hospital bed wondering what I can do to convince all those big politicians that it's a lot cheaper to find a cure than to pay for all of this medical treatment. I mean—hasn't anyone told these guys that a stitch in time saves nine?"

"Maybe," I suggested, as I put the form down, "women with breast cancer should organize themselves to march topless on the heads of governments—you know, to all the Parliament Hills, White Houses and Palaces of Justice."

"Now *that* would get some attention," she agreed, laughing now. "Women like me who can't walk could be pushed in wheelchairs or on stretchers."

"We could put brown bags over our heads."

"No," she said, "people need to see the anguish."

"Maybe," I continued, "maybe women shouldn't be wearing prostheses. Maybe we should be more visible."

Her eyes suddenly darted around the ambulance. "If we hit one more bump I'm going to spew," she warned.

I slipped a basin underneath her chin before she vomited green-black bile. When she was finished, I washed her face off with a cloth.

"That's better," she said, leaning her head back against the pillow. "It's all comfort now," she explained. "My treatments are just to try to make me comfortable."

Her eyes had teared up. She made a deep sighing sound and said, "What a terrible way to die."

I nodded, unsure what to say. I took her hand in mine and held it while we rode in silence the remaining few blocks to the Cancer Agency.

The next day was hot and beautiful. Other than at Donna's luncheon, Deirdre and I hadn't seen much of each other. But she called that morning and suggested, "Let's go kayaking." We agreed to pack food that could be shared, and both of us turned up at the beach with a bottle of champagne.

It was the middle of the afternoon when we set off. We paddled for about an hour towards an island and then slipped along its shoreline, following a pair of kingfishers as they flew low over the water. The wake from a ferry almost swamped us, the island itself rising from the water like a breaching whale. When we reached an isolated bay, we hauled the kayaks onto the rocks. A few seals plunged back into the ocean, alarmed.

I felt very pleased with my right arm and shoulder. I had expected them to protest much more than they had. Managing the tiring repetitiveness of paddling had been one of the hurdles in my recovery.

Deirdre went ahead, carrying the paddles and food to a comfortable rocky ledge where she set out our small banquet: bagels, smoked salmon with red onion and cream cheese, Greek olives, pickles, brie and grapes. We popped the first of the champagne corks and leaned back against a log that must have drifted away from a boom. The water was so still we could see fish jumping. We talked about what tasty morsels they might be after, and Deirdre made some fish movements with her mouth. It made me laugh.

There was still a lot of heat left in the late afternoon air. As we ate, the sky began to darken. The colour of the water changed with the deepening sun. The surrounding islands appeared farther and farther away. We both kept saying, "We're losing light, we should be going," but we couldn't motivate ourselves to move. The water was so flat and beautiful, the air so still.

After we had finished both bottles of champagne, it seemed like a good idea to go swimming. For a time, we just floated around bathing in the red light of the water and letting the buoyance of the ocean hold us up.

It was dark when we finally slipped the kayaks into the night water. We made an agreement not to discuss what time it might be until we hit shore. We joked about how long it had been since we'd gotten into trouble together. It was obvious that Deirdre had decided to handle our previous difficulties by acting as if they had never happened. Maybe that's the smartest thing to do, I thought. Maybe she's right.

Under a full moon rising, we paddled across the water, moving in and out of each other's reflections, awed by the iridescence falling from our paddles.

"Do you know what causes it?" Deirdre asked.

"Who cares?" I sighed, possessed by the moment. "It's just so beautiful."

As we moved almost soundlessly towards the shore we could see the beams of hand-held flashlights scanning the water surface like feeble searchlights.

"Oh, God," Deirdre said. "They're out in numbers."

My eyes searched the water. "I'm just glad I haven't seen any rescue vessels around."

"You know," Deirdre said, "if our kids did this to us, we'd kill them."

"It's kind of like riding a bike without a helmet, isn't it?"

"Uh huh."

As soon as we were within calling distance, we heard the outraged voices of our daughters. "You guys, what if a boat ran into you … you didn't even take a flashlight … why didn't you tell us you'd be so late?"

I blinked a small ineffective light that I always carried with me when I went kayaking.

"Like, a lot of good that would have done you," Jenny said.

"Better than nothing," I said hopefully.

Deirdre and I looked for our husbands, relieved to see that they weren't there.

"What? No men looking for the drowned loved ones?" she asked.

"They're at home," a reproachful voice said. "They figured you would turn up sooner or later."

"Ta-da! And here we are," Deirdre sang out as she jumped onto the beach.

I smiled to myself. For my daughters, breast cancer had no longer been the threat.

The next day, as I went back to see Shannon, I noticed a few dark clouds collecting in the distance. On the way to the hospital I stopped at a gift store and picked up a frog similar to mine. I placed it on Shannon's lap. "It's a cancer-cell eater," I informed her.

Even at this stage of the disease, she was thrilled. "Well, he can have a feast if he stays with me," she said, dangling his long legs this way and that. Suddenly she mimicked the frog and said, "Croak." We laughed.

Her husband, Martin, had been sitting with her. He decided he'd walk their dog while Shannon and I had a visit. He looked grateful for the break.

As soon as he had left, Shannon said, "I had a dream. It was a waking dream."

"Tell me," I prompted her.

She spoke slowly, looking past me. "I was surrounded by blackness. Like an ocean. My body was full of pain. Terrible pain. Everywhere. I gave myself up to the blackness and, as if I were in a movie, I watched myself die. And then the darkness turned to light. Somehow, it was a turning point for me. Kind of a letting go. Now I feel … well, I feel okay about dying. What do you think about that?"

"I think maybe it's telling you something about life."

"I can't imagine not being. Can you?"

"Maybe there's no such thing as not being."

Briefly, she made eye contact with me, and I could see she was waiting for me to say something more. As if I'd given it previous thought, I went on, "Maybe we're just held here a brief time by the planet's motion and then—" I paused "—and then we go somewhere else."

Her husband walked back into the room with their dog, Beau. Beau acknowledged me briefly, then bounded straight onto Shannon's bed and burrowed under the covers. I left the room with the sound of her laughter in my head.

I didn't get back in to see Shannon for a week. I was stunned by the change I saw in her, but I was determined not to show it. She looked up oddly from beneath the hospital sheet like a child surprised at having been found where she wasn't supposed to be. Her skin had a transparent look, the light sepia of an old photograph. It was as if some part of her had already gone.

I leaned over and placed a kiss on her forehead. I recognized a smell that both attracted and repelled me, holding me there. I couldn't shake it off. It was the smell of death.

I placed my hand gently over hers. "Shannon?" I said quietly.

When there was no response, I sat down and took her hand in mine. I listened to her laboured breathing for a long time. Eventually her husband came in.

I stood up, gave Shannon's hand a squeeze and left.

I walked out of the hospital and stood on the sidewalk just to feel the air on my skin. I heard something. I looked up into the blue sky and saw Canada geese heading south, steering by planets or God knows what, and I thought that maybe, somehow, Shannon had left on some other unexplainable journey.

Driving home, I put the radio on scan and was bombarded with irrelevant phrases and bits of music until I heard a woman say, "That's the thing … there are no magical solutions for breast cancer." The interview was drawing to a close. The radio announcer asked, "Can you imagine a world where all women have only one breast? Can you imagine a world without women?"

I decided to stop off at Pat's. I didn't want to be alone. Pat knew where I'd been. She hugged me tightly.

"I doubt she'll make it through the night," I said.

We walked out onto the deck, listening as more geese flew overhead. Some of the leaves had turned, but most of them were still hanging on.

I slumped down into a large deck chair. "Remember when I used to be fun?" I asked her with the faintest smile.

She smiled back. "But you still are—it's just that you've had some challenges of late. You were brilliant at Donna's."

Thunder rumbled in the distance. Surprised, we both looked up at the sky. Clouds that had hung there in the windless air all day had started to close in. The hot dry spell would soon be over.

"I have to try to do something, Pat," I said. "I have to do something about this disease for my daughters, your daughters, Deirdre's ... for all our daughters."

"Then I consider it done," she said.

I gave Pat an appreciative hug. Walking out to the car, I almost collided with a raccoon herding her progeny across the driveway and up a tree. Their dark forms stood out against the sky—a mother and babies in the safe high branches.

A few days later I browsed through a newspaper at work. It was there at the back: "TAYATA, Shannon Leslie. Passed away peacefully on Friday...." How strange, I thought, reflecting on Shannon's battle—how strange to say that she passed away peacefully, though I knew in the end it had been that way.

I was still staring blankly at the paper when Deirdre dropped by the station to say hello. "What're you reading?" she wanted to know.

"The obituaries," I said. "Amazing how a person's life changes. I never used to read the obituaries."

"Someone you know?" she asked, sitting down in a nearby chair.

"Shannon. A woman who had a mastectomy a week before me. She didn't make it."

"That must be hard on you." She paused and then added, "Others who don't make it."

I met her gaze. "Deirdre, I've started to write a book about breast cancer—"

"Oh, no," she almost shrieked. "A book." She slunk lower in the chair, starting to laugh. "Please don't put me in it."

"Do you mean that? I have to know. You've been such an important part of my life."

She picked up a small pillow and clasped it closely to her, staring at me curiously for a long time with her wide, lively eyes. I heard a tiny whine in the air—the soft, steady insistence of a mosquito.

Her fingers stroked the pillow. I wondered if she was thinking of her mother, or maybe her daughters.

"Go ahead," she said finally. "This is a book that needs to be written."

When I got home, the red cedar walls of the house glowed with the light of the setting sun. I was happy to find everyone in the family there. Peter wore a cowboy hat. He'd been away again, stopping off for a visit at his uncle's ranch long enough to bring home a hat and lasso. Right now, he was busy trying to rope a dining room chair.

"You better watch out," I warned Freyja.

I went over to Peter cautiously and lifted his hat so that we could give each other a respectable embrace. For the first time, I noticed a few grey hairs near his temples. I gave them a gentle tug. "I'm working on my Gary Cooper look," he told me.

Jenny exploded into the room, tripping on the top step of the stairs. She ended up sprawled on the floor. Freyja decided it must be a game and dove right in. In the middle of Jenny's shrieks I shouted, "Jenny, it's too bad you weren't born on a planet where there isn't any gravity."

Katherine came upstairs, calling ahead, "What on earth is happening?"

"Oh, look at Katherine," I said, stepping over the writhing mound of arms and legs on the floor to give her a hug. It was the first time I had seen her in her ambulance uniform.

"I'm very proud of you," I said, stepping back to admire her polished look.

Jenny was still on the floor, complaining, "Hey, I'm the one who's injured. I'm the one who's supposed to get the hug."

I tousled Jenny's hair with my hand and said to Peter, "Just look at Katherine, will you? Our biggest baby."

"You can't talk like that if we work together," Katherine warned.

"I won't, I promise. It will be all professional."

"I'm glad you're so confident," she replied. "I'm having nightmares about being at some horrible accident scene and hearing myself say: 'Help, Mommy!'"

I laughed. "Call me what you used to—Moz. Remember? You can't take the Mom out of Roz."

"Are you actually working?" Peter asked her.

"No, I'm riding shot-gun," she said, staring strangely at her father in his cowboy hat. Having finished her courses and passed her exams, Katherine would now go along as a third crew member or an apprentice.

"What ambulance are you working tonight?" I asked.

"The skids," she answered.

I churned up a face. "Well, one evening of that will be worth about a year of university. Now remember: never stand in front of a door, watch your back, always make sure you know where the exit is, don't lean against anything, double glove, watch for stray gunfire. There are rats the size of terriers—"

"Moz, give me a break," she broke in, laughing.

We all went to the door to see her off. The first few drops of rain had started to fall, lifting the scent of the forest into the air. I wrapped my arms around Jenny, who stood in front of me.

"Katherine, you need a rain jacket," I called as she went down the stairs.

"I don't have one yet."

"Wait." I grabbed my uniform raingear from beside the door and threw it down to her.

"Thanks, Moz," she called.

The others went back inside, but I watched until the red taillights of her car disappeared around the curve below the house. A lot of things had been taken away from me in the past months. But a lot of things had been given back, too. I had what I wanted. The normal rhythms of the family were restored.

And tomorrow would be another day. A new morning. Life was full of endless possibilities, and I was eager to live as fully as I could for the rest of the sweet life that was given to me. Because now I was not dying of cancer—I was living with it. I knew there might be challenges ahead. But then, I've always liked adventures.

Afterword

Imagine yourself picking up the newspaper one Saturday morning to find a front-page headline screaming, "747 crashes. All 415 passengers killed. Onlookers shocked and horrified."

Unrolling your paper over morning coffee four weeks later, you read another huge headline: "Second 747 crashes. No survivors. Families and witnesses stunned." Now imagine that this same headline appears every month for a whole year. One month it appears twice.

Of course, the situation would never get to that stage. Before it did, every 747 in the world would be grounded. There would be public inquiries. Those responsible would be called to account, and heads would roll. International aviation would not be the same until the problem was solved.

This year, 5400 Canadian women will die of breast cancer—the same number as would perish in those thirteen imaginary plane crashes.

In 1994, 16,300 Canadian women will receive a diagnosis of breast cancer. In other words, every day this year, forty-five women will tell their workmates, friends, families and lovers that they are in a life-and-death struggle with breast cancer. For these women, it will be like stepping onto an airliner knowing that there is a serious mechanical fault in the engine. They'll hope and pray that repairs will hold long enough for them to reach their destination of a full life span.

Just how big is the social and economic impact of this epidemic of breast cancer? Throw a pebble in a pond for every woman who is diagnosed, placing the breast cancer patient at the epicentre. The shock to each of these women cannot be overestimated. Over 80 per cent of us who develop breast cancer have no family history of the disease, and over 70 per cent of us have no obvious risk factors other than being women who are growing older. No one is safe, not even men, who represent almost 1 per cent of all breast cancers diagnosed.

Further out from the centre are ripples representing those who are affected closely but indirectly. Each new diagnosis carries with it a clutch of people who are forced to deal with the disease by association. How many people in your life would be shaken to the core if you told them today that you had breast cancer? Business understands that the cost of days lost due to illness, low office morale and death goes beyond money. To consider breast cancer as only a women's issue is narrow, cold and incredibly short-sighted.

For each woman, encountering breast cancer is a 3-D, technicolour experience. Nobody leaves the breast cancer theatre without being terror-stricken, no matter what outward appearances suggest. Physically there's an indelible reminder that our lives have been put in peril, that breast cancer pursues us. And we are also grieving the loss of our belief in our bodies. Through no action of our own, they have betrayed us, and we face the future knowing that the sword of Damocles hangs over our heads.

Our reactions to this threat on our lives register everywhere on the emotional scale. Some women need to withdraw and lick their wounds in complete privacy. Rosalind MacPhee shed tears only from one eye, wetting half of her face for days on end. She wept silently when bodily fatigue and the weight of dealing with the disease rubbed her nerves raw. Rosalind held on with a quiet sadness, trying to protect her family from her anguish. She never expressed anger or deep fear except in her dreams.

Some of us have high-decibel responses. After one of my radiation treatments, an offhand remark made by my teen-ager prompted uncharacteristic fury. A heavy glass and brass floor lamp was standing beside me when I saw red, and I picked it up from the base and smashed it against the floor. Sparks flew, glass shattered and the brass fittings broke apart as I threw the twisted base across the room. It felt good. If I was out of my mind, it was the right place to be. I also cried—loudly and often—at Puccini, Oprah, the dog, newspaper articles and, once, at an African violet I was unable to nurse back to health.

What is it about this illness that prompts such reactions? As adults, we often take our ability to control our actions and manipulate the world around us for granted—until it is threatened. After my diagnosis, I had the terrifying feeling that I had no more influence over my destiny than a back-seat driver in a runaway car.

Information is the key to regaining a sense of control. Yet so much of it is controversial and conflicting. Almost every day the newspapers, radio and TV bring us tantalizing and confusing bits and pieces about breast cancer. Gene therapy hopes. Clinical trial scandals. Cures based on radical diet approaches. Mammography controversies. Debates over pesticides and high-voltage wires. For the layperson it's almost impossible to separate fact from fiction.

The family doctor is usually the first stop for a woman who has questions about a change in her breasts. Eighty per cent of all lumps are not breast cancer. But it's important for any woman to know that her family doctor may only see one or two new cases of breast cancer in a year. I have sat in on many breast cancer support groups, and I am convinced that too many diagnoses are delayed due to the doctors "Watch-it and Follow-it" of the world. A breast change, whether it be a lump, a nipple discharge or a variation in shape, skin colour or texture, always warrants immediate investigation. I have always respected intuition. If a woman feels that she has a serious problem, she is most likely right. Only a woman can feel her breasts from the inside out!

If you have a worrisome lump or change and your doctor suggests watching it and following it, assertiveness on your part is absolutely necessary. The change should be investigated through mammography, ultrasound and/or some form of biopsy. If cancer is detected after you have insisted on active follow-up, you may have gained a head start on treatment. If the biopsy turns out to be negative, celebrate.

If you are diagnosed with breast cancer, take a deep breath. Take two. Rosalind MacPhee discovered that she had probably been host to her tumour for years. Realize that you do have a week or two to get through the initial trauma, figure out what questions you want answered and consider your options.

You may be tempted to look for the fastest way just to get rid of the cancer, but the decisions you make now will be with you for the rest of your life. Take some time. There is no such thing as a stupid question. Make a list of all the questions you have and make sure you get answers. Under stress, information is difficult to absorb, so you may need another set of ears at your appointments. If you cannot bring someone else with you, a tape recorder is useful, and written notes will be invaluable later on.

You have a right to more than one opinion on your diagnosis, and treatment options and opinions about them may vary. For example, many studies have confirmed that lumpectomy is just as effective in treating early breast cancer as mastectomy, yet there are still wide regional variations in the type of surgery performed. If you need more than one expert to educate you on the disease, you must have it. When your life is at stake, only the best medical expertise available to you will do. Understanding and choosing what will happen to you makes it easier to come to grips with whatever results the treatments may bring.

When you are faced with the terrifying diagnosis of breast cancer, accurate information specific to your own medical situation is currency for life. But information is not always easy to locate in the form and language needed. Rosalind MacPhee had access to the B.C. Cancer Agency library and the expert, willing direction of the librarians there. She avoided the trap of becoming paralyzed with information overload.

We should all be so lucky. When I was told that I had breast cancer, my mind buzzed with static. I was devouring supermarket tabloid advice and compulsively reading brochures my doctor had given me without absorbing anything. This in spite of the fact that I have a degree in library science and a background in teaching "learning to learn" skills to corporations.

My reaction was a common one. As Rosalind MacPhee queried, what must it be like for those of us who find reading difficult, who need translation into our mother tongues, who are unaware of how to find even the most basic materials and have to depend on others for our information? What must it be like for those of us who live in rural areas, miles from any cancer treatment centre? There need to be more cancer treatment clinics, and these clinics must offer counselling services that can help patients and their families with both emotional and informational needs.

In time the static faded, making it possible for me to learn and, like others, I have become an expert on my own case.

Many people are surprised to find out that each woman's breast cancer has individual characteristics that direct treatment. Breast cancer is not a single disease, but many diseases under one name.

The emotional impact of breast cancer unfolds over time. The amount of tissue removed does not always relate to the level of anger, grief and sadness felt by a woman at diagnosis, during treatment and for the rest of her life. Many of us who are diagnosed experience the loneliness of the long-distance patient. For a few intense, terrifying weeks, we—or our cancers—are the centre of attention, but radiation and chemotherapy can drag on for months leaving us running on empty.

We have no choice but to learn to live under conditions of uncertainty. We carry with us the fear of a truncated future because we know that even with the earliest diagnosis, the fiercest treatments and the best prognosis, no one can give us a guarantee that breast cancer won't kill us. We long to return to "normal," but it doesn't take long for most women to realize they must restructure their lives and values to develop a new definition of normal life.

Initially, Rosalind MacPhee appeared driven more by a need for action, through researching her disease, than for emotional support. However, after the immediate crisis had passed, accumulated stress brought her to her knees and to the door of a grief counsellor. Not everyone has access to a safe and confidential place to express her loss and grief, but I pray that every woman who must deal with cancer finds a compassionate person willing to listen time and time again to her story.

People often wonder how to help someone else. You may be the most important person in the life of a woman undergoing breast cancer treatment, or you may be an acquaintance who wants to help out in some small way. Whatever you can give, commitment is the key. An offer to help is the first step, but more than a "call if you need me" is appreciated. Be proactive. Suggest what you can and would like to do.

Gail, a single, working mom, lives a two-hour ferry ride from Vancouver with her three kids. Her cancer required surgery and intensive chemotherapy at the B.C. Cancer Agency in the heart of Vancouver. She needed help. Her friends and work-mates held a potluck supper strategy session to plan what to do. One woman moved in with the kids on the days when Gail had to be in Vancouver. Others did basic house repairs so Gail could have the option of selling her home quickly if she needed to, and one friend helped her put her finances in order and write a will. For years Gail had eaten a macrobiotic, organic diet. One person took on the task of delivering the food Gail needed to keep her spirits up to the hospital kitchen, where it was prepared daily. This same friend also became Gail's gatekeeper, protecting her from unwanted advice and issuing health bulletins to the team.

Currently there is nothing we can do to prevent breast cancer. We can't butt out, buckle up, wear a safety helmet or get inoculated. We can't slap on a sunscreen or slip on a condom. No wonder we react with frustration. A dozen years ago the chances of a woman developing breast cancer over her lifetime were one in thirteen. Today her chances are one in nine. Mortality rates have remained essentially the same over the past two decades. Diagnosis and treatments are improving, with more battles being won. The war, however, is spreading.

Why hasn't a cure been found? Money is part of the prob-lem. From the June 1992 federal government report "Breast Cancer: Unanswered Questions," the Canadian public dis-covered that of the approximately $52 million put into cancer research by government and the private sector in 1991-92, only $3.1 million could be identified as dollars targeted to breast cancer research.

As a result of intense lobbying by advocacy groups, the federal government has since raised its research contributions to $20 million, spread over five years, and has challenged the general public and the corporate sector to match funds. It's a start, but the funding is still paltry in relation to the money given to other diseases.

We tend to be impatient with research and, by extension, researchers themselves. However, researchers are no different from most Canadians. They have car payments to make, kids' teeth to straighten and groceries to buy. Like most of us, they can afford to turn their attention, skills and intellects only to projects likely to be funded. Large research projects take sustained finances to set up, run and evaluate. In short, research goes where the money goes.

I cannot help but believe that if there were enough money in the pot for targeted breast cancer research, there would be more minds willing to focus in that direction. We need to pay for the best brains available to work for us, and we shouldn't be afraid to ask for results. Perhaps it's time to set national policy on the nature and direction of cancer research. After all, targeted research placed the first human on the moon.

The priority for breast cancer research should be prevention: we need to find ways both to stop the disease from developing in the first place and to prevent the women who already have the disease from dying. Until we have a way of preventing breast cancer, we look forward to increasingly sensitive, accurate screening developments.

If it is true that we harbour breast cancer for up to a decade before diagnosis, then how many Canadian women are walking around today with tumour time-bombs in their bodies?

Currently, mammography is the most reliable tool we have; it can pinpoint tumours from two to five years before they can be felt. The debate over screening mammography, which offers mammography to healthy women without any symptoms of the disease, rages internationally. There is agreement that women over fifty and women with a family history of the disease will benefit from screening. What is in dispute is whether a diagnosis from mammography before age fifty will extend life and catch enough cancers to make it worth the money spent. And even though women today are living longer lives, those of us over the age of sixty-nine are not actively encouraged to utilize screening programs everywhere in Canada.

I do not see any good reason for waiting any longer to make screening mammography readily available to all Canadian women. It took over twenty-five years for cervical cancer screening, in the form of today's Pap smear, to become a standard feature of our health care. It has been responsible for saving thousands and thousands of Canadian women's lives. I believe that screening mammography programs will have the same pattern of success.

Like the Pap smear, mammography isn't 100 per cent foolproof. Rosalind MacPhee's tumour wasn't picked up by X-rays. I know other women whose doctors located their cancers. My own tumour, though, was missed both by my own breast self-examination and my doctor's efforts, yet was located on a regular mammogram.

Breast cancer is about life, and saving it. With or without breasts, life, love, sex and femininity can carry on. However, if women believe that breast cancer always means losing breasts and then dying anyway, there is precious little encouragement to check their bodies regularly. It is important for women to know that finding breast cancer in its early stages offers a far, far better chance of cure and of saving our breasts, with less need for chemotherapy. My early diagnosis and medical situation allowed me to choose a lumpectomy, which has left a very insignificant scar. Those who have had more extensive surgery and want reconstruction will find that it comes in many forms.

Most breast cancers are still found by women themselves, through chance. A slippery hand feels a lump while soaping up in the shower. A lover notices a change in skin colour or texture. We may increase the odds for early detection by adding a physician's clinical breast exam, mammography and breast self-examination to our yearly and monthly routines. We need to know the normal geography of our bodies.

For generations breast cancer has been considered too embarrassing and too horrible to speak about. Those of us with the disease have had to confront the fact that breast cancer alters or amputates our breasts and challenges basic beliefs about femininity, nurturing and sexuality. Our relationships may change. Our jobs may be threatened. There are still whispers that breast cancer is contagious. Is it any wonder that we have been hiding our breast cancer scars in the closet?

Advocacy offers a means to channel our energies and to do something positive about a disease over which we have had precious little control. We know that silence and denial can kill. Advocates work on many fronts to break silence and shine an uncompromising light on all the issues surrounding breast cancer.

Recently breast cancer has become a hot news item. Advocacy groups have emerged, mad as hell that so much more money has gone to other diseases and unwilling to accept peanuts any longer. Our population is aging, with more women falling into the higher-risk categories. The political establishment has been surprised by the overwhelming public attention paid to the 1992 all-party parliamentary subcommittee hearings on breast cancer. The media has found new, dramatic fodder for readers and viewers.

This is fertile ground for action. Advocates are beginning to recognize that breast cancer cannot be "sold" on facts and figures alone, and that one of the most powerful tools of advocacy is the telling of personal stories. Awareness and influence are created by gut responses to human events as well as logic. Whether or not we have breast cancer, the impact each of us can make by speaking out in public forums and in committee rooms can be great.

Education about breast cancer is crucial and must begin early. If our daughters can graduate from high school knowing how to roll a condom on a wooden penis, why couldn't they be taught how to feel their own breasts as part of a normal routine? Teen-agers are not generally at risk for breast cancer. However, I have met enough women in their twenties and thirties with the disease to know that no one is immune. Had these young women been doing routine breast self-examinations, they might have been alerted to changes in their breasts that turned out to be cancers.

On the political front, finding champions to fight for your issues in parliament is one of the advocate's greatest challenges. Contact your local MP's office to ask for a list of parliamentary standing committees and their members. Among these MPs you might find someone who will take up your issue.

Write to your MP and request a meeting. Form a delegation, and ask for specific commitments when you meet with your MP face to face. Outline the content of your meeting in a follow-up letter and send it by registered mail to the MP. Send copies to other appropriate people as well. Long before election time, create a questionnaire, the same for all political parties, asking candidates about their views on funding, support, or whatever your delegation considers most important. Wave their answers under candidates' noses in public when the media has the cameras running.

Research dollars are allocated on the federal level, but support for cancer centres and medical services comes from provincial governments. Use the same tactics with them. Ask in writing about the waiting lists for radiation treatment. Ask what support services for breast cancer patients are offered by social services departments. Get commitments.

Never, ever underestimate the power of the consumer and the corporate world's need for good public relations. Ask corporations what they do with their charitable money. Educate them on the severity of breast cancer. Find out how many women work for them, and then figure out how many of these women will be affected by breast cancer over their lifetimes. When you see products that are aligned with a worthy cause, give that company your business. If you don't need or want the product, you can still send a letter of appreciation to the president and the board of directors. Advocacy is an energetic, optimistic activity—and optimism is healthy.

Sitting in support groups over the years I have heard two statements consistently: "Breast cancer is the best thing that's ever happened to me" and "Breast cancer is the worst thing ever to happen in my life." It can be both at the same time. When one piece of a life puzzle alters its shape, inevitably everything else shifts. Friends adjust, bolt, move closer or quietly drift away. Families can pull together or fall apart. Rarely have I heard women delighted to be labeled "survivors," and more than one thesaurus has been well thumbed in the search for an alternative way to describe ourselves.

However, surviving breast cancer is the first step. After that, I hear women say that they want to live a full life. For many, breast cancer has been a wake-up call.

After very difficult breast cancer treatment, one woman I know decided to risk everything, to give up her job and spend her savings to live out her dream of becoming a diver in the South Pacific. When breast cancer recurred with a vengeance, she declined further treatment that would do her little good. Instead, she camped in the wilderness with her beloved father and visited friends. She felt satisfied with her choices and intends to continue to live her life to the very end still "calling all the shots," as she put it. Whatever our individual priorities are, Sue's example speaks to all of us. As she says, life is not a dress rehearsal.

Finally, where there is life, there is hope. And there's a lot of life in women who have survived a bout of breast cancer or who have gone several rounds with the disease. There's dedication in the physicians who work with us on a daily basis and in the researchers who desperately want their efforts to make a difference.

All of us need to become involved. As women and men; as family members, partners and friends; as activists, educators and fund-raisers, we need our best thinking and most determined optimism to bring to the task of wiping breast cancer from the face of the earth. In Rosalind MacPhee's words, "Women have got to stop thinking that if they avoid learning about the disease, they'll avoid the disease itself." We must all deny denial.

Judy Caldwell
President
Canadian Breast Cancer Foundation, B.C. Chapter

For information on breast cancer issues, fund-raising, lobbying, education and patient support services, contact the following groups:

Canadian Breast Cancer Foundation, National Office, 620 University Avenue, 7th floor, Toronto, Ontario M5G 2C1, (416) 596-6773, info line: 1-800-387-9816

Canadian Cancer Society, National Office, 10 Alcorn Avenue, Toronto, Ontario M4V 3B1, (416) 961-7223

Breast Cancer Action, Billings Bridge Plaza, P.O. Box 39041, Ottawa, Ontario K1H 1A1

Provincial Screening Mammography Programs: Every province is different. Call local telephone information services and cancer treatment centres for mammography screening availability in your area.